J MARTIN LITTLEJOHN
An Enigma of Osteopathy

Dedication

This is dedicated to Rory, Salvador, Phoebe and Oona who have taught me much during the sunset years

Also to my dear friend, Robin Kirk (1939-2014)

J MARTIN LITTLEJOHN
An Enigma of Osteopathy

By John C. O'Brien MA DO
National Osteopathic Archive, London

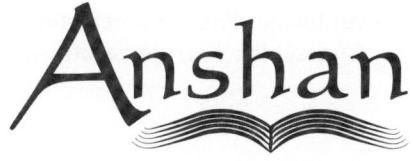

JOHN MARTIN LITTLEJOHN
An Enigma of Osteopathy

By

John O'Brien

Published by:-
Anshan Ltd

6 Newlands Road
Tunbridge Wells
Kent. TN4 9AT

Tel: +44 (0) 1892 557767
Fax: +44 (0) 1892 530358

e-mail: info@anshan.co.uk
web site: www.anshan.co.uk

© 2016 Anshan Ltd

ISBN: 978 1 848291 386

All rights reserved. No part of this publication may be reproduced, stored in a retrieval system, or transmitted in any form or by any means, electronic, mechanical, photocopying, recording or otherwise, without the prior written permission of the publisher.

The use of registered names, trademarks, etc, in this publication does not imply, even in the absence of a specific statement that such names are exempt from the relevant laws and regulations and therefore for general use.

Every effort has been made to trace all copyright holders, but if any have been inadvertently overlooked the publishers will be pleased to make the necessary arrangements at the first opportunity.

British Library Cataloguing in Publication Data
A catalogue record for this book is available from the British Library.

Copy Editor: Andrew White
Cover Design: Emma Randall
Cover Image: Phoebe Greenwood
Typeset by: Kerrypress Ltd

Contents

About the Author	vi
Preface	vii
Acknowledgements	xi
List of Abbreviations	xiii
J Martin Littlejohn Timeline	xv
Chapter 1 The Early Decades: Birth, Adolescence and Adulthood 1865-1898	1
Chapter 2 The Kirksville Years 1898-1900	23
Chapter 3 The Chicago Years	39
Chapter 4 Those Degrees, Doctorates and Visits: Return to Britain	53
Chapter 5 The House of Lords Select Committee Hearing 1935	73
Chapter 6 The Gloaming Years 1936-1947	87
Chapter 7 Finale	101
Addendum	113
Index	117

About the Author

John O'Brien practised as an osteopath for 40 years. In that time he also taught osteopathic history and clinical studies (although not continuously), including spending 21 years as a final clinical examiner. He gained his MA in the History of Medicine and, recently, has been co-founder and archivist at the National Osteopathic Archive in London.

Preface

My interest in this physically slight but giant European influence, John Martin Littlejohn, first arose some 50 years ago, inspired by Colin Dove, who was at the time the History and Principles of Osteopathy lecturer at the British School of Osteopathy. This controversial man, (JML not Colin!), appeared to invoke praise and criticism in almost equal measure, a sort of osteopathic Jekyll and Hyde character. Transatlantic sources spoke about a romantic tryst with Blanche Still, dark stories of strife, a vendetta with A T Still's family, and a recurrent pattern of dispute with the American osteopathic profession and more specifically, his Chicago colleagues. A chastened JML returned to Britain, eventually founding his own teaching establishment, the BSO, maintaining its survival almost singlehandedly for two decades, before disaster occurred.

Many of his British colleagues perceived him as a martyr, sacrificed on the altar of the House of Lords select committee hearing of the Osteopaths Act in 1935 by Sir William Jowitt KC, British Medical Association chief Counsel. This event rather postponed UK osteopathy from seeking further statutory regulation for nigh on sixty years.

How will the profession now react to any criticism of a hallowed being from these pages? Where does the truth lie between the two extremes of his reputation?

A number of colleagues have attempted to write a biography of Littlejohn, but my version has utilised historiographical methods to try to discern wishful material from more authentic documents. Would using these techniques and degrees of analysis give a more transparent image or metaphorically, muddy the waters even further? I had some advantages though: the National Osteopathic Archive had collected much early material relating to JML which has helped enormously in shaping thoughts on his personality, his resoluteness, his obstinacy, his osteopathic ethos and his legacy, both professional and familial. I was fortunate to have known two eminent academics who helped me understand the nature of historical research, Professor Sally Mapstone, Pro-Vice Chancellor of Oxford University, and Dr Elizabeth Hurren, my illustrious History of Medicine Masters supervisor. In order to understand JML's complexity, I am fortunate to live in a rural idyll with its capacity to be separated from human contact for days at a time. This has afforded me undisturbed periods for study and research. When one reached an impasse, a prolonged walk in the countryside would often clear the air.

Although much has been written of JML, in the process of writing this book a number of questions would constantly arise. One of these was the important understated role played by his younger brother, James Buchan Littlejohn, who has had a greater influence in the destiny of American Osteopathy. James not only brought major surgery to the American School of Osteopathy (ASO) Kirksville, Missouri, but also its permanent presence as a specialisation within the ASO curriculum, together with obstetrics. On moving to Chicago, James co-founded the American College of Osteopathic Medicine and Surgery, with major surgery as a crucial part of the college curriculum when it became a further year's extension course. Moreover, ACOM & S undergraduate training included the controversial teaching and prescribing of drugs, even after threats from the American Osteopathic Association to withdraw accreditation for doing so. For certain, James Buchan was in the vanguard of exhorting the profession to progress towards full medical licensing, an eventual outcome being the reform of the osteopathic schools into regular medical institutions (1936-1960). He was an inspired lecturer and bore few grudges, not even towards those who had treated him disreputably, unlike JML who found it difficult to let bygones be bygones. Unfortunately, a schism between the brothers in 1913 was never to be healed. One hopes some day that James's contribution will be recognised in the pantheon of Osteopathy, perhaps someone out there in Illinois will write a suitable biography too?

Another recurring theme to ponder is why six osteopathic medical schools survived when all the remainder within the Flexner Report of 1910, under the chapter "Sects", vanished so abruptly? Was it to do with osteopathy's locality within newly fledged Midwestern states? Did rural communities produce excellent practitioners, perhaps less academic but more practical and sociable? Why did these educational establishments proliferate further into 30 schools of osteopathic medicine?

Returning to JML, his was a distinguished academic record, a golden student who effortlessly accomplished so much while attending the acclaimed Coleraine Academical Institute and Glasgow University, aged just 16 years. This scholastic ability met its nadir when he entered the portals of Columbia College, New York to take his PhD but failed, it became his dark night of the soul. He appears from that time onwards to accept his demise by collecting fourth rate doctorates, at the same time enjoying the respect and company of lesser academic folk.

JML's adult life witnessed great changes from his first vocation as a nonconformist Presbyterian minister within an ever-increasing nationalist Catholic Ireland: his American citizenship with the twin backdrops of the near annihilation of the indigenous peoples, (especially in the Midwest) and the USA's unassailable rise as a de facto world power - a youthful mighty country able to export not only its vast agriculture and prodigious commerce but also its culture: JML's return to a Britain on the verge of war, the emergence of the Labour party as a national force at the expense of the Liberals: the aftermath of the First World War would see the elimination of European imperialism, the rise of Nazi Germany and Soviet Russia, and the gradual erosion of the British empire at the expense of American hegemony.

One hopes that this book will throw light on some of the inconsistencies and controversies surrounding JML, including the setbacks in his life. His wife Mabel and children gave him stability during these times, although they rather resented the BSO and its students monopolising his time and financial generosity at the expense of his own family. But without his total commitment, the school would have closed.

Whilst this book disregards some details felt to be irrelevant, it is by no means seen as a definitive work on JML, but, hopefully, should add to our knowledge and understanding of the man.

Acknowledgements

There are a number of people I wish to thank for their assistance. First and foremost is my friend and colleague, the late Robin Kirk, who always provided stimulating discussions. All his friends still miss those occasions around a table when Robin would provoke interesting debate. A year ago his premature death gave me notions of my own mortality and the impetus to finish this project. I owe much to Reverend Drew Gregg of Creevagh Presbyterian Church for his unfailing help in gleaning JML material from different sources concerning his time as a Presbyterian minister; Chris Campbell entered in a light hearted debate over JML's Presbyterian ministry, thanks to him for allowing me access to his considerable research into JML's early life; Dr Martin Collins for his diligence in preserving much JML material at the British School of Osteopathy ; Dr Jorge Esteves and Dr Ollie Thomson of the BSO research department offered spirited discussion over some considerable time; special thanks to Audrey, Lady Percival, who advised me on the BSO during the late 1940s and early 1950s; Margery Bloomfield gave me infinite support and humour; Sara Kennard, her mother Ann plus cousin Michael Newman gave me much help in sorting out some of the Littlejohn family complexities; Lee Sands, BMA archivist, provided much help over the select committee papers (1934-5); During my travels in USA, thanks are due to staff and librarians at the Chicago College of Osteopathic Medicine; officers and archive staff of the American Osteopathic Association, downtown Chicago; also, Jason Haxton, Debra Lagouda-Summers and staff at the Still Museum of Osteopathic Medicine, Kirksville. Thanks to all at the National Osteopathic Archive History Society; Charles Hunt and staff at the BSO; Nick Harding and fellow BSO clinic tutors; to my grand daughter Phoebe who produced this wonderful JML cover portrait, with the tiniest of help from her mother, Anna Greenwood; Many thanks to Emily Wainwright for her cover design; Andrew White, my publisher, copy edited the project with gusto and good humour; and finally, Sue Wainwright who as usual, has always been there to provide patience and encouragement.

John C O'Brien MA DO

ABBREVIATIONS

ABO	Association of British Osteopaths
ACOMS	American College of Osteopathic Medicine & Surgery
AMA	American Medical Association
AOA	American Osteopathic Association
ASO	American School of Osteopathy
BA	Bachelor of Arts
BCh	Bachelor of Surgery
BCC	British Chiropractic College
BCN(O)	British College of Naturopathy (& Osteopathy)
BD	Bachelor of Divinity
BMA	British Medical Association
BNA	British Naturopathic Association
BS	Bachelor of Surgery
BSO	British School of Osteopathy
CCO	Chicago College of Osteopathy
CCOM	Chicago College of Osteopathic Medicine
DD	Doctor of Divinity
DO	Doctor or Diploma of Osteopathy
ENT	Ear, Nose & Throat
FRS	Fellow of the Royal Society
FRSL	Fellow of the Royal Society of Literature
FSSLA	Fellow of the Society of Science, Letters and Arts
GCRO	General Council and Register of Osteopaths
GOsC	General Osteopathic Council
HoL	House of Lords
IAO	Incorporated Association of Osteopaths
LCO	Littlejohn College of Osteopathy
LCO	London College of Osteopathy
LCOM	London College of Osteopathic Medicine

LLB	Bachelor of Law
LLD	Doctor of Law
LSOC	Looker School of Osteopathy & Chiropractic
MSO	Manchester School of Osteopathy
MB	Bachelor of Medicine
MD	Doctor of Medicine
MP	Member of Parliament
MRO	Member of the Register of Osteopaths
OAGB	Osteopathic Association of Great Britain
PhB	Bachelor of Philosophy
PhD	Doctor of Philosophy
WSO	Western School of Osteopathy

Time Line of JML: A life on the high road, toil and vale of tears

1865 15 February John Martin Littlejohn born 27 Taylor Street, Glasgow.

1870 Family move to Seil Island: JML enters Easdale school, Seil Island.

1877 Family move to Garvagh, Northern Ireland; JML attends Garvagh Scientific Academy (1877-79) graduated with 1st prize.

1879 attends Coleraine Academical (1879-1881) Reformed Presbyterian Church Scholar: Intermediate Education Board Ireland honours and prize (1879-1880); prizes cum laude: Classics, English & Science (1879-1880-1881).

1881 enrols Glasgow University (1881-5) Reformed Presbyterian Church Scholar, undergraduate arts course: 1st Class in Classics, Mathematics, Logic, Metaphysics, Rhetoric, Moral Philosophy; English language & literature; Scholar in mathematics; Tutor at University (1883-5); Divinity (1884-5); 1st class honours and university prize in Mental Philosophy; special university prize in Oriental languages but does not attend graduation ceremony. Also attends part time Original Secession Seminary (1884-6).

1885 attends Reformed Presbyterian Seminary, Belfast, NI (1885-6): ordained 7th September 1886.

1886 accepts the living of Creevagh, County Monaghan (1886-1888); lectures in Theology & Sacred Literature at Ballybay Union Hall; resigns his living, summer 1888. May have taken living as locum in Shropshire.

1888 returns to Glasgow: brother James attends Anderson's Medical School, and JML may well have attended lectures unofficially. Has a serious fall outside the Faraday Laboratories.

1889 following brother William's emigration to USA, JML convalesces in New York and attends Columbia College. He graduates belatedly from Glasgow University as MA (1889); enrols in Bachelor of Divinity (BD) (1889-90) gaining 1st class honours and the Henderson prize in Theology – *Thesis on Sabbatism of Hebrews IV 9 (1891)*; Member of Glasgow University Council (1889).

xv

1890 Glasgow University Law School (1890-92): LLB with honours; Special prize in Feudal and Scottish Law; University prize in Constitutional Law, History and Conveyancing; and William Gold medal in forensic medicine. Law member of students' representative council (1891-92) Taught at Rosemount College (1890-92).

1892 Columbia College, New York: fellow of faculty of Political Science in Political Philosophy, *The Political Theory of the Schoolmen and Grotius* for PhD (1892-1893); research as student in cathedral and university libraries of England, France, Germany, Switzerland & Italy (Summer1893); never completes his thesis and viva voce exam at Columbia; illness takes him to Waukesha, Wisconsin; enrols as student at postgraduate school of Theology, National Night University, Chicago (1893-94).

1894 National Night University, Chicago: Doctor of Divinity (DD) *The Christian Sabbatism* dissertation (1894); and PhD for thesis, *The Political Theory of the Schoolmen and Grotius* (1895); Christian Add-Ranx University, Waco, Texas- Doctor of Law (LLD) 1894; Amity College, Iowa, President (1894-97).

1897 resigns Amity College. Enrols at National Night University in National Medical College course (1897-98); visits A T Still for treatment at Kirksville.

1898 suspends medical course to join American School of Osteopathy (ASO) Faculty as Professor of Physiology (1898-1899); JML officiates with his father at brother David's wedding to Mary Forbes (sister of Bill Smith's wife) in Kirksville; Lecture to Society of Science, Letters and Arts (SSLA), London "*Osteopathy in Line of Apostolic Succession with Medicine*".

1899 JML appointed ASO Dean.; at SSLA, Crystal Palace, South London, July, gives lecture "*Osteopathy as a Science;*" attends sister Elizabeth's (Bessie) marriage to Tom Anthony in Ipswich, and introduced by Bessie to Mabel Thompson, his future wife. Dismissed as ASO Dean after 5 months, to be replaced by Hildreth; Bill Smith summarily sacked and the three Littlejohn brothers (JML, James and David) allowed to continue on faculty until the end of the academic year.

1900 death of father James, buried in Kirksville cemetery; leaves Kirksville July, returns to Chicago: renews medical course at National Medical College which has been absorbed into Dunham Medical School. JML with David and James co-founds American College of Osteopathic

Medicine & Surgery (ACOMS) 405, West Washington Boulevard, Chicago. Another LSSA lecture, *"Osteopathy: A new view of the Science of Therapeutics;"* marries Mabel Alice Thompson, in Ipswich, England; returns to Chicago to settle at Lake Bluff; President of ACOMS, lecturing in Physiology, Principles and Therapeutics.

1902-4 graduates from Dunham (MD, Dunham) cum laude: Dunham assimilated with Hering Medical School; enrols at Hering and lectures in Physiology; MD Hering (1904); Hering and Hahnemann medical college merge (1904); Professor of Applied Physiology, Hahnemann. ACOMS: transfers to 495-7 West Monroe Street; merges with the American College (1903); brother David resigns to concentrate on public health medicine.

1905-1909 JML starts to outline his greater osteopathic concepts; James and JML plan to raise standards to include Materia Medica and full state medical subjects; ACOMS changed to Littlejohn College of Osteopathy (1909); Professor of Applied Physiology, Hahnemann (1904-6); President of Associated Colleges of Osteopathy (1908-1910); A T Still Research Institute: researches into neoplasms (1908).

1910 Littlejohn College of Osteopathy (LCO) unable to gain full state licence for graduates. Flexner Report - highly critical of all eight osteopathic colleges but LCC specifically criticised as 'an undisguised commercial enterprise'. Final failed attempt to meet the State Board of Health by expanding Materia Medica and Pharmacology course whilst AOA threaten to withdraw accreditation for adding drugs to the curriculum; Materia Medica and Pharmacology dropped: all efforts abandoned for Littlejohn College to be recognised as a medical school. JML's views on an expansive osteopathic lesion rejected wholesale by the profession.

1911-12 LCO adds fourth year to the course. In 1912 senior members of LCO faculty meet with brother James to plan reorganisation; the AOA is critical of Flexner Report: JML's mother Elizabeth dies in Chicago, buried with her husband James in Kirksville cemetery.

1913 LCO assets sold by the Littlejohns to a group of Chicago osteopathic physicians to run the newly named Chicago College of Osteopathy as a traditional DO school; JML applies for headship but loses to brother James: JML irreconcilable at the outcome, leaves the USA with Mabel and six children and renounces his American citizenship. Purchases Badger

Hall, Thundersley, Essex;. Opens a practice in Piccadilly, London and Thundersley; joins the British Osteopathic Society, associated with the AOA (later to become British Osteopathic Association in 1915).

1914-21 Has the practice transferred to 48 Dover Street, London and two satellite practices in Enfield and Thundersley. The British School of Osteopathy (BSO) incorporated (1917); Noel Buxton MP in the House of Commons extols the virtue of Bonesetting and Osteopathy for assisting the war wounded; death of A T Still.

1922 BSO finally starts at Dover Street practice; JML Dean; Sir Herbert Barker, knighted for his Bonesetting, is appointed BSO director.

1924 Wilfrid Streeter inaugurates the Osteopathic Defence League (ODL)

1925 The BSO moves to Vincent Square; JML is BOA President (1925-6); BOA manifesto outlines role of osteopathic manipulation and training in the UK; first two BSO graduates join BOA; JML leads a delegation to hand in letter to Neville Chamberlain MP, Minister of Health.

1926 successful BOA inspection of BSO with the proviso to transfer BSO ownership to an independent BOA board of control; last attempt by BOA for BSO mandatory ownership; BOA countermands BSO accreditation and membership to BSO graduates; JML resigns as BOA president and his BOA membership; BSO graduates form Association of British Osteopaths (ABO); death of William Looker.

1927 12 Looker students taken on at BSO; exploratory talks with Incorporated Association of Osteopaths (IAO) for further training and study at BSO (1927-8); George Bernard Shaw opens BOA clinic,

1928 Looker students graduate at BSO; talks with staff and students of defunct Western School of Osteopathy and its sister, British College of Chiropractic in Plymouth to transfer to BSO.

1929 IAO takes over the BSO alumnal ABO to form the largest association of UK trained osteopaths.

1931 W M Adamson MP introduces private members Bill (failed); BOA attempt to gain a Royal Charter.

1933 Bob Boothby MP introduces private members Bill (failed).

1934 Osteopaths Bill passes its first reading in the House of Commons and referred to a select committee at the House of Lords (HoL); British Medical Association set up committee opposing Bill.

1935 March - Select Committee meet; JML witness for the Bill but responds inadequately; supporters of the Bill try to stop proceedings, citing the founding of a voluntary osteopathic register; September - the HoL select committee report severely criticises JML and the BSO.

1936 Setting up of General Council and Register of Osteopaths (GCRO); IAO changes name to Osteopathic Association of Great Britain (OAGB).

1937 First and second tranche of BOA members join GCRO en masse; OAGB and non-member BSO graduates boycott GCRO.

1938 GCRO executive persuade OAGB executive to join GCRO individually; first tranche of OAGB members, non-member BSO graduates and a number of BOA members en masse.

1939 GCRO inspection of BSO; BSO gains accreditation; Further tranche of OAGB members and non-member BSO gradates join GCRO en masse. OAGB and non-member BSO graduates hold majority on GCRO; GCRO BOA members decline; JML retires from teaching at the BSO, citing failing health; JML in talks with GCRO officials to sell his BSO shares.

1940 JML sells his majority control of the BSO; de facto running of BSO left to Shilton (Webber) Webster-Jones and Clem Middleton; it remains open during London blitz bombing.

1943 JML appoints Jocelyn Proby as deputy Dean but Proby wishes to return to Ireland and recommends T Edward Hall to replace him; Webber and Middleton retire in protest.

1944 Death of Edgar Littlejohn (son) in India; JML's health declines further.

1945 Death of Charles Lief, BSO graduate (son of Stanley); BSO reopens; JML very frail.

1946 T Edward Hall resigns as BSO vice-Dean; opening of BOA London College of Osteopathy; founding of British College of Naturopathy.

1947 JML congratulates Webber on his appointment as vice-Dean of BSO; JML dies.

xix

Chapter 1
The early decades: birth, adolescence and adulthood (1865-1898)

A small, slightly built, rather complicated individual, in latter years somewhat stooped in posture with a characteristic shy, diffident air, John Martin Littlejohn was unable to converse with small talk, chatter or gossip. However this rather physically insignificant individual had a profound influence on osteopathic development throughout the first part of the 20th century. He had no charisma as a showman nor a sense of humour to lace his dry lectures, normally essential qualities required for leadership. Also, he could be obstinate, vague and ill focused on the matter in hand. Mild in nature, difficult to rouse to anger or to an emotional outburst, but his tenacity in guiding his school and his generosity to the students were outstanding.[1] Although he died some 70 years ago, his influence continues to cast a shadow over osteopathy today.

How did a bright young man, respected and esteemed by many, but held in derision by others, become such a controversial figure in osteopathy?

This is the story of his remarkable journey: through good times and bad; through both successful academia and also somewhat doubtful attainments; his catastrophic appearances during the select committee of the House of Lords in 1935; and his sheer dedication through thick and thin. We must go back to the beginning of the story, his birth, to discover how John Martin Littlejohn became such a controversial person.

J Martin Littlejohn (JML) was born on 15th February 1865 at 27,Taylor Street, Clydebank, a northwest suburb of Glasgow, Scotland, adjacent to the river Clyde. His parents, James, a son of a collier, and Elizabeth, a daughter of a handloom worker, had eight children in total. John Martin was fourth born, only five survived into adulthood.[2] Previously, in November 1863, their eldest son, Buchan aged 6, and eldest daughter, Janet Elizabeth aged 5, both died, within a week of each other, from scarlet fever - a deadly and highly contagious streptococcal infection brought on by a combination of poor diet and unpasteurized milk.

1

Scarlet fever epidemics seemed to occur in cycles of 5-6 years and poor nutrition corresponded to the high price of wheat during these periods.[3]

> *"The age group most vulnerable to death by illness was the very young. Deaths of children under ten accounted for more than half the deaths in Glasgow in the early 19th century, and even as late as 1861 some 42% of all deaths in the city were in this age group. In Scotland as a whole, the Registrar General's first annual report in 1861 found that the highest proportion of deaths occurred in the age group under five years."*[4]

The youngest daughter, Margaret, died aged 18 months in 1873 at Kilbrandon, West of Scotland. Subsequently, William, the third born, in 1862, became the eldest surviving child, followed by JML and 2 years later by James Buchan. Additionally, Elizabeth Alexander, their only living daughter, was born in 1869 and five years later, the youngest, David.

What their parents may have lacked in financial resources they made up by providing a secure, protective, enquiring and loving environment. James Littlejohn was a clergyman within protestant nonconformist Calvinism, the Reformed Presbyterian Church (RPC). His impecunious state was balanced by a resolute determination, fortified by his faith.

This RPC had its origins within dissenting religious sects hostile to King Charles 1 and his successor, Charles II, during the Civil War.[5] These religious protestant groups had made a covenant with Parliamentary forces, hence the term "covenanters". It disassociated itself from the Church of Scotland in 1690 and later, in 1876, merged with the Free Church to become the United Presbyterian Church.[6] James Littlejohn's training had required attendance at Theological Hall, Glasgow, scholarship being an essential part of his ministerial training. Subsequently, he scratched a lowly paid living acting as a probationary preacher, locum and peripatetic minister to congregations around Glasgow and surrounding towns without a regular clergyman.

In 1870, James accepted a post taking him and his family to Lorne near Oban, on the west coast of Scotland. The congregation comprised of 51 Gaelic-speaking members who were expected to pay for his employment.[7] It was a difficult position: the minister was expected to work very hard attending to their spiritual and social needs while in reality the congregation took a firm grip on things as paymaster. It was a

Chapter 1

tricky balance for all concerned, a similar situation that J Martin would experience some two decades hence. What we do know is that James' spiritual territory covered the area of Seil and Luing Islands together with the mainland town of Lochgilphead.

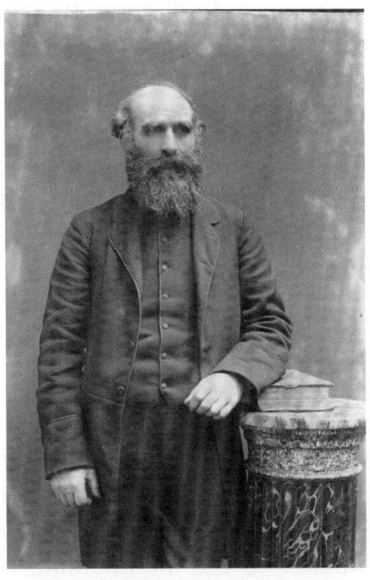

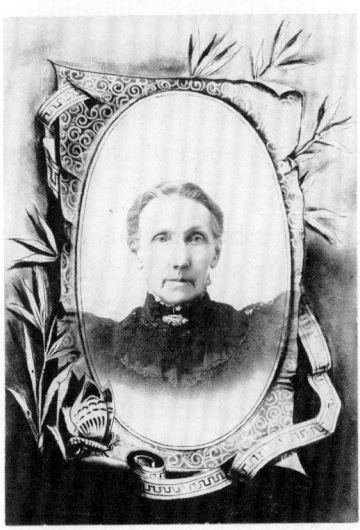

James and Elizabeth Littlejohn, parents of JML

These small scattered Reformed Presbyterian communities spread over 40 miles distance extracted as much value from their ministers as possible on the lowliest of stipends. James Littlejohn rose to his task with vigour, determination and fortitude. The family settled in Ardencaple Cottage on Seil, probably located adjoining the substantial Ardencaple House. The cottage consisted of 5 rooms, and the Littlejohns employed a maid to help with household chores.

It was not long before stirrings among the majority Reformed Presbyterian Church (RPC) Synod, an assembly of ministers and church elders, sought unification with the Free Church (known as "the Wee Free"). Previously, James had supported a minority synod and had, initially, left the Wee Free to join the RPC. He was loath to support such a motion.

A year later, his opposition had come to the attention of the church elders. More significantly, only 16 out of his local membership backed his disapproval to the merger. Although his post became untenable while holding his views, he gallantly agreed to remain in place until a new incumbent was appointed.[8] Moreover, this episode did not appear to weaken James' faith or resolve. During this three-year interregnum he continued to administer to the membership until unification took place at the Kilbrandon Free Church. Nonetheless in 1876, there were sympathetic members in its more vibrant and wealthy sister Church in Ireland who welcomed his reputation for exemplary behaviour and firmness of faith by offering him a living in Garvagh, Northern Ireland. Perhaps significantly, his acceptance of a lowly stipend provided further evidence of his suitability.

Meanwhile, his son JML was building his own reputation as a bright scholar at his Easdale primary school, an education which contained the Classics: Greek and Latin, together with mathematics and physics. His parents provided an academic atmosphere at home, which contributed to all the children's schooling. J Martin easily outpaced William (his elder by three years), a difficult situation that William faced throughout his teens and early twenties.[9] Much information about J Martin's early years has been gathered from his curriculum vitae (CV) of 1894 attached to his Columbia College dissertation. Its accuracy has been questioned but parts of it can be verified as authentic from Glasgow University records.[10]

Be that as it may, in 1877, James took up his living in Garvagh, Northern Ireland.

Chapter 1

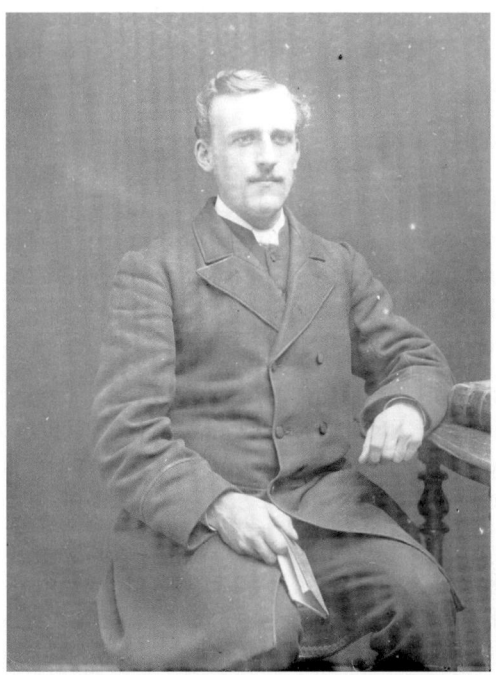

William Littlejohn as a young man

Garvagh, from the Gaelic, meaning 'rough place or field', in the county of Derry (Londonderry), is situated 11 miles south of Coleraine, with the river Agivey flowing through, it is celebrated for its salmon and trout fishing. The area surrounding the town offered highly productive farmland, far superior to that around his place of work back in Scotland. It was a staunch Protestant market town famed for the Battle of Garvagh in 1813, when a force of 400 Catholic tenant farmers and their supporters were repelled from storming a tavern known for holding meetings of the local protestant Orange Order. This conflict was heralded as a great victory among the Protestant community, to which RPC members were party, its place in Northern Ireland history was indelibly marked.[11] Accordingly, James Littlejohn was seen as a man to recognise and preserve such traditional enmity among a small but steadfast congregation.

Meanwhile, JML's scholastic achievements were affirmed further when he went to Garvagh Academy, winning first prize for topping his class, and a year later, he gained honours and a prize in his Intermediate Education

5

Board exams.[12] His intellect was clearly blossoming and, significantly, he was awarded a RPC scholarship in 1879 to join the upper school at Coleraine Academical Institute.[13]

Both William and JML were boarding at the Institute, a voluntary grammar school acclaimed for its academic record and its sporting achievements throughout the whole of Ireland. The headmaster (1870-1915) T G Houston was a Covenanter member of the Ballyclabber RPC for 24 years and presumably therefore immersed in that particular theological outlook. Thus it is likely that he would have been kindly disposed towards both boys.[14]

In JML's final school year (1880-1), he gained three prizes: Classics, English and Science.[15] Significantly, he rather outclassed William once again, aged 18 years, by being awarded a place on the same theological course at Glasgow University at the same time as his elder brother.

JML and William both intended to follow their father into the ministry. The university course included a broad first and second year curriculum, embracing mathematics, metaphysics, oral philosophy, logic, through to English language, English literature and Classics. During this time, JML developed his intellectual ability further, collecting first class honours and the University prize in Moral Philosophy in 1883. By the following year, he specialised in divinity, mathematics and natural science, while continuing with general subjects. Subsequently he and William attended the Original Secession Seminary, Glasgow (1884-1886) to hone particular nuances, tenets and tracts specific to the Covenanters' creed, under the auspices of the Northern Presbytery, the most powerful administrative province of the RPC in Ireland.[16] JML was awarded first class honours in his University finals and a special University prize in Oriental languages.

These prizes and grades are quoted from his CV, but official records do confirm his attainments.[17] Much has been written concerning his failure to officially graduate, specifically his reluctance to attend the university graduation ceremony to take an oath of allegiance to his alma mater. It is suggested that the RPC and its sister denominations might abhor any oath of allegiance, according to covenanter tradition, especially to crown or country. There is an alternative explanation, namely that provided he had "ticket" evidence of completion of his course, the cost of ceremonial attendance was not worth paying. Indeed, a significant number of graduates concluded exactly those sentiments, irrespective of dissenting religious values. This covenanter anti-establishment refusal to take any official oath is an early demonstration of JML's rebellious nature, as seen later with his unflagging support for osteopathy being "outside the pale" of orthodox medicine.

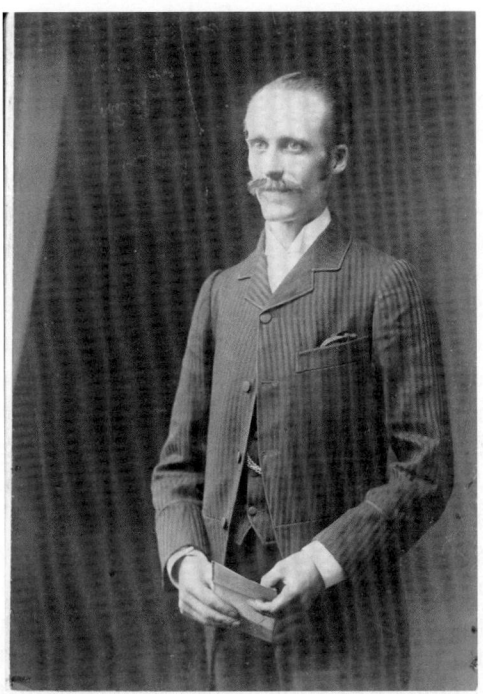

J Martin Littlejohn as a young man

Be that as it may, his family and the RPC authorities would have been delighted with his intellectual progress, because academic achievement was highly regarded among the RPC hierarchy. His confidence in his own academic abilities must have been gained earlier during his time at Garvagh Academy and Coleraine Academical Institute, then later by four years study at Glasgow University. His arrival, with William, at the RPC Seminary in Belfast, appeared to be the culmination of their continued desire to join the ministry. The course at the Reformed Presbyterian Theological Hall, to give its formal title, had two professorial chairs, Systematic and Pastoral Theology, including church history and Hebrew. This postgraduate course was held over a winter semester of 4 months duration.[18] At the same time he wrote a series of articles for *'The Covenanter Magazine'* which would also add some weight to his potential career prospects among the list of expectant probationary ministers awaiting a locum position, peripatetic ministry or a fixed regular livelihood. JML did not have to wait long in 1886 before he received notice from the Southern Presbytery of the RPC. The Creevagh Presbytery congregation outside Ballybay, county Monaghan "had secured a comfortable manse and raised their stipend to £110.00". [19] [20]

JML, aged 21 years, must have been delighted at his appointment to a congregation of 200 members, made up of a rural community of self-sufficient, hard-working tenant farmers, their families and farm workers. It was, on the face of it, an ideal opportunity for a young, ambitious, gifted minister to make his mark.[21] What appeared as a straightforward prospect however was considerably more complex for one so naïve and inexperienced. Surely his father's own experience of being exploited with poor financial reward and questionable security of tenure among the RPC Lorne congregation in the West of Scotland would have been discussed? Alongside this, was James's continued lowly stipend from the wealthier Northern Presbytery RPC in Ireland an equally significant factor in his son's recruitment? James's counsel must have been sought by both sons, and crucially before JML's acceptance of the living at Creevagh. James would have cautioned him on its lowly stipend, but balancing this argument was the opportunity to gain experience and utilise it as a stepping stone to further his career. Moreover James, and to a lesser extent both sons, were well aware of the historical nature of the 'geo-political' climate existing in the province of Ulster.[22]

What would have been prevalent in the Littlejohn family discussion was Creevagh's situation: a well-known but well-off Protestant covenanters enclave, surrounded at best by an indifferent, and at worst, a hostile Roman Catholic populace presided over by a Pope, "old red socks", the great protestant antichrist. Meanwhile, its location within County Monaghan was one of three counties, (the others being Cavan and Donegal) with Catholic majority populations, out of the nine counties constituting the province of Ulster. Littlejohn family conversation would have reflected on Catholic ascendancy in these three counties. Ironically, Southern Irish Protestants had been in the forefront of Irish Nationalism, Irish culture and the Irish Language. The subsequent rise of all these among Ireland's majority Catholic population during the nineteenth century caused considerable anxiety within Northern Ireland Protestantism, especially those of Presbyterian provenance. Specifically, the most vulnerable being those in minority Ulster Protestant communities surrounded by

Catholic majorities. Family conversation would have centred on local Catholic aspirations favouring maintenance of the Irish language and a flourishing Gaelic Athletic Association reviving the sports of handball, hurling and Gaelic football. More ominously under discussion would have been the spectre of Irish nationalism in its guise as the Irish Republican Brotherhood or Fenians, financed and led by Irish Americans. Consequently, these exposed minority communities, especially their Presbyterian ministers, their families, manses and church buildings, felt themselves as potential targets of an alien people with differing religion, culture and language.

Moreover, JML would duly have noted that apart from the Reverend Thomas Cathcart (1806-1857), no minister had held the Creevagh living for very long. This might suggest the transitory nature of the minister's prospects and reality of his situation. JML would have little knowledge of the mind-set of the congregation prepared to withstand a Catholic majority. This stalwart Scottish settler covenanter stock could be suitably unimpressed by preaching of an intellectual ethereal nature. Its kinship was sustained by a nonconformist, down to earth, fire and brimstone, dyed in the wool anti-Catholic tradition.[23] In their perspective, any preacher worth his salt would need to fuel this collective ardour as a bastion against Irish nationalism, an united Ireland and Catholicism. Woe betide a minister not adjusting his views to those of his congregation or not kowtowing to its needs either.

JML accepted the invitation, even though the living included a modest "raised stipend of £110" and a "comfortable Manse". Perhaps this latter description of the house was not accurate, because a year later J Martin appealed for funds to raise money for a new presbytery. Grudgingly this was acceded to by the congregation, possibly a decisive enough reason why so few ministers had continued serving Creevagh.[24] Be that as it may, his incumbency was celebrated on Tuesday 7th September 1886 in the presence of his family. Whatever his reservations, he assumed his ministerial duties as well as initiating theological lectures in the nearby Ballybay Union Hall.[25] This latter role might have been important for JML's long term plan to be enacted as a career move to a more liberal, educated congregation within a majority protestant Ulster county or an academic position elsewhere. His suitability among the Creevagh worshippers was not helped by his youthfulness, and his inexperience, neglecting necessary time for making regular visits to the sick and individual calls to his congregation. His youth, intellectual credentials and esoteric ramblings appeared misplaced among congregation members. Moreover, he seems not to have consulted his elders or congregation on matters they considered of mutual interest. These traits conveyed a less than attentive, somewhat distant minister neglecting his primary duties of service to his people.

Things appeared to deteriorate fairly rapidly after a fundamental disagreement concerning his failure to visit the sick and infirm; his lack of stewardship to inform and consult his congregation; a boat trip to Liverpool; and permission from the Southern Presbytery of raising funds for a new manse which appeared to have mixed support from the congregation.[26] JML's stipend was very low and accordingly he might have thought that the manse fund was a flexible source of money for him to withdraw certain expenses without informing church elders. Perhaps some of it was used for expenses on his trip to Liverpool. This venture was supposedly authorised by the Southern Presbytery, with the purpose of collecting further funds for the manse project. However, his journey might also have included an opportunity to reconnoitre a vacancy in Shropshire.[27] After his return to Creevagh, his congregational elders confronted him with "certain difficulties in their financial position" and "supposed irregularities with their pastor". He stated that he had used funds for expenses as authorised by the administrative office of the Southern Presbytery, which had given permission for him to travel to Liverpool and raise money for the manse. He failed to satisfy his church elders or produce evidence of any funds collected or provide travel confirmation from the Southern Presbytery. They accused him of causing financial difficulties and certain irregularities. Consequently, a significant number of the Creevagh congregation refused to pay anything towards his stipend and threatened to leave the church. Serious complaints were made to church leaders and more specifically to the Southern Presbytery.

It was one of the elders of Creevagh, attending a meeting of the Southern Presbytery, JML himself being absent, who enquired whether the RPC authorities had sent JML to Liverpool with a recommendation to collect money, and had the Southern Presbytery sanctioned a new manse? The Clerk of the meeting informed the elder that no such order had been given for a trip to Liverpool, but the Creevagh presbytery recommendation for a new manse had been authorised. The clerk then read minutes from the previous August meeting concerning a new manse and a recent letter received from JML. Consequently, during the meeting, matters were considered while other Creevagh elders demanded answers. It was decided to refer all these complaints to a special future meeting at Creevagh in a month's time.[28]

On the 6th March 1888 the meeting took place, among those attending was his father James. Two elders and two members spoke of their complaints against their pastor. Afterwards, a unanimous decision was made: no insurmountable difficulty had arisen; the congregation must consider their pastor's youth, inexperience and show Christian charity towards him; and finally, JML must demonstrate magnanimity and be prepared to consult, respect and seek approval from his congregation in the discharge of his ministerial duties.[29]

What the meeting failed to convey was a complete breakdown of relations between a minister and his congregation, neither party was prepared to accommodate the other, especially a congregation which had totally lost the confidence in its pastor through his laissez-faire behaviour and his economy with the truth over his trip to Liverpool.

Moreover at the next meeting in May, a Creevagh elder adamantly stated that nothing had been resolved and, if anything, things had worsened. As evidence he provided a list of complaints signed by 82 members, which stipulated their wish to terminate JML's Creevagh ministry forthwith. It was agreed that the matter should be transferred to the Synod meeting at the end of the month. Moreover, Creevagh members should not sever their connection with the church but desist from any talks encouraging dismissal of their minister. In the meantime, another clergyman would take over all pastoral duties and be responsible for settling all existing difficulties.[30]

At the next synod meeting a member of the Creevagh congregation, favouring a more charitable approach, produced a minority report listing support and approval for its minister. However, the newly installed temporary cleric in charge of Creevagh presented a more forthright picture of the majority feeling, namely an outright rejection of JML, full stop. Dismissal was the only way forward now. Accordingly, the Moderator decreed that taking all things into account, sympathy should extend to both parties in dispute. Clearly, peaceful negotiations had failed. He declared that it was the duty of the local church to decide a course of action and for the synod not to interfere. In these circumstances, he continued, the local church should not condemn, impugn or denigrate their pastor but release him with a generosity of spirit. Not withstanding the Moderator's intervention, JML immediately resigned his ministry, but requested that his name be placed on the roll of Southern Presbytery ministers and not put back on the probationers' list.[31]

How had things gone so wrong for JML in less than two years ministry? Was this placement a poisoned chalice from its inception?

Between 1857-1928, no minister had lingered long at Creevagh. Five years' would elapse between his dismissal and another regular incumbent. Perhaps the RPC Southern Presbytery had exploited JML's naivety and his inexperience by recommending this living within a besieged community, smartened by a particular ideology. The church authorities were hypocritically indecisive at the synod meeting because they and also the Creevagh congregation knew that power lay with the congregation alone. It was the arbiter of JML's fate. It paid his stipend and could withdraw its own corporate or individual membership at any time. (During these sessions, the Moderator might well have looked enviously at the hierarchical control within the Catholic church over its members and wished that he could intervene more effectively.) However JML continued to preach to two further congregations and petition the synod for outstanding monies owed by the congregation to him. Southern Presbytery authorities washed their hands of the affair by declaring no further liability necessary.[32] The Creevagh congregation must have felt that JML had forfeited any compassion, compensation or surplus pay by his furtive behaviour. However, there were other strands to this event.

Records show that both brothers James Buchan Littlejohn and JML were domiciled at Munslow, Craven Arms, Shropshire, but also that JML had been a minister there.[33] It is said that his brother William became its minister and that his brothers were merely making fraternal visits. As suggested earlier, could this have been the reason why JML had made the trip to Liverpool to investigate the possibilities of taking up a post?[34]

This episode had future ramifications for the Littlejohn family. JML had been used by the authorities to provide spiritual succour to a stoical protestant Creevagh congregation which had clearly demanded much more during his tenure. Other sources mentioned rumours concerning JML's unwanted interest in three unmarried ladies within the congregation. (Perhaps this could be the "certain irregularities with the pastor" mentioned in the Southern Presbytery papers?) One year later, William Littlejohn had had enough. He had seen his father and brother suffer under the difficult political climate in Ireland, while he himself no longer wished to endure the softer political climes of Shropshire. He emigrated to the USA. And five years later the rest of the family followed.

Father James retired from his post at Garvagh in early 1893, but JML, far from quitting the idea of a religious career, had decided to reenter Glasgow University to resume his studies, whilst younger brother James began his medical training at the university.

During this particular four-year period (1888-1892) of his life, JML's biography is quite difficult to construct. Possibly he may have been pursuing a number of different opportunities, including mathematics and physics, connected with the Faraday Laboratories at the university, headed by the great Sir William Thomson, later Lord Kelvin.[35] However, chronic ill health rather overcame any plans when he fell on concrete steps outside these laboratories, fracturing his skull, leaving him unconsciousness for four hours.[36] His health deteriorated further from bouts of chronic haemorrhages of the throat, probably caused by the Epstein-Barr virus producing glandular fever, common to all universities. Similarly, symptoms caused by streptococcal infections of the throat producing chronic tonsillitis were commonplace at the time. He consulted Dr Matthew Charteris, sometime Professor of Clinical Medicine at Anderson's medical school and Professor of Materia Medica at Glasgow.

Charteris probably recommended his colleague, Sir Morrell MacKenzie, a specialist of the larynx who had famously treated Crown Prince Frederick of Germany for a supposed benign laryngeal tumour the year before. The following year, the prince ascended to the imperial throne as Kaiser Frederick III, only to die from an undiagnosed malignant tumour of the larynx, much to the fury of his excellent German medical staff. A book, *The Fatal Illness of Frederick the Noble* was published, outlining the mistakes made by MacKenzie, who was censured by the Royal College of Surgeons for this misdemeanour.[37] He wasn't effective with JML either, who continued to suffer intermittent attacks for a number of years, but Charteris and MacKenzie did recommend convalescence in America, in order to recuperate.

While William had emigrated to America in 1889 principally to join the Pittsburgh Presbytery, his brother JML, suffering from poor health, also sailed to New York, specifically resting in a sanatorium on Long Island.

We have no proof of them travelling together or meeting up, having voyaged separately.

JML appeared to have made intermittent trips to Columbia College, perhaps with an eye to studying there more permanently.[38] However, he returned to Glasgow and at some stage took an official oath of allegiance at a graduation ceremony to receive his Master of Arts (MA) for his original coursework (1881-1885). Meanwhile younger brother James continued his medical training and there is a probability that J Martin was attending some of John Gray McKendrick's masterly physiology lectures at the same time too. He might have been one of those students who are attracted to subjects others are pursuing, the grass being greener so to speak.

J Martin's appetite for knowledge at times appears as a mass confusion of facts in his writings - he loses the thread of his thoughts and direction but somehow restores it some pages further on. This waywardness blights a lot of his writing throughout his life and applies to his career too. It appears that he had too many options, being attracted to medicine, teaching, and of course continuing his religious studies. Finally, he decided to read Divinity, which included a dissertation as part of his studies. In 1891 his thesis on "The Sabbatism of *Hebrews IV: 9*" was awarded the Henderson Fellowship Theology prize of 20 guineas, retrospectively.[39]

At this stage he favoured another alternative to medicine, namely law. This suggests he rejected the notion to continue a religious vocation by turning towards a career in the legal profession. He supplemented his funds by teaching at Rosemount College, a ladies' establishment in Glasgow. A teaching experience he rather enjoyed.[40]

He embarked on a general Bachelor of Law degree at his alma mater, graduating cum laude in 1892. He further dallied with James' medical course, clearly attracted to physiology by McKendrick's inspiring lectures, but he enjoyed teaching too. The young, full of potential 16-year-old freshman of 1881 had now become a professional, rather aimless mature student of 27 years, enjoying his time as law representative on the student council and joint editor of the *Glasgow University Magazine*. Furthermore he continued to do well academically, picking up a university medal in Jurisprudence, a special prize in feudal and Scottish Law and a university prize in Constitutional Law, History and Conveyancing. This was all most worthy academically but in practice he lost all notion of a legal career.[41] Consequently, J Martin Littlejohn's thoughts turned back to America, his family over there: a new start, a new direction.

By the fall of 1892 JML had registered as a Ph D student in the faculty of Political Science at Columbia College, New York. It was a prestigious institution, having been founded in 1754 as King's College, after King George II. Thirty years later, following the War of Independence, its name was changed to Columbia. By 1896 the college was renamed Columbia University. Its expansion into graduate faculties in political science, philosophy and pure science placed Columbia in the higher echelons of American postgraduate education.[42] JML was indeed fortunate to have found such a respected institution and faculty. Meanwhile, he had pondered on the subject of his thesis prior to leaving Scotland, and had been heavily influenced by the life and works of the late Sir James Lorimer (1818-1890) with the help of Lorimer's former pupil, William Galbraith Miller, JML's lecturer in Jurisprudence at Glasgow.[43][44] In the acknowledgements of his printed unpresented PhD dissertation he pays tribute to Lorimer, Miller and Reginald Lane Poole, fellow of Jesus College, Keeper of the Archives and lecturer in Diplomacy, the University of Oxford. [45] JML probably met him during his European research tour of summer 1893, Oxford having an outstanding tradition for welcoming and assisting others during their research stay in the city.

Quintessentially, the basic tenets of PhD strategy are firstly choose a topic which is not open-ended, and secondly select your supervisor wisely. If either of these factors is at variance with these rules, then beware. Unfortunately, JML decided on *"The Political Theory of the Schoolmen and Grotius"*, its very title being rather grandiose and vague. Hugo Grotius, a jurist of the Dutch Republic, was a founder of International Law, basing his reasons on so-called ' Natural Law". He was also a protestant theologian whose ideas resonated with Calvinists.[46] A schoolman was "master in one of the schools or universities of the Middle Ages who was versed in scholasticism; scholastic".[47] This European connection meant that JML would at some stage need to return to Europe to research extensively. Not only that, was he able to limit his subject matter? Like a number of JML's propositions, one cannot help but think that it was doomed from the start. However, by either luck or good judgement, his supervisor at Columbia was magnanimous, the indefatigable William Archibald Dunning.

Dunning had graduated from Columbia University in 1881. Five years later, he was appointed to teach history, including Political Science. He continued to do so until 1903, and was awarded a professorship in 1904. Dunning had a reputation for relevant, meticulous research (although JML dedicated his dissertation to him, one cannot help but speculate how JML's slightly scatter-brained approach must have tested the patience of his supervisor).[48]

Dunning was probably relieved to see JML leave for his grand tour of medieval libraries of England, France, Germany, Switzerland and Italy during the summer of 1893.[49] On returning to the USA from his travels, JML realised the enormity of his task. Moreover he still reverberated the dry, understated reflection of such a commitment given by Poole during his stay in Oxford. JML's enthusiasm, dedication and positivity to even write up his thesis were severely compromised. Throughout his past troubles his undoubted scholastic ability never let him down, but he was challenged by this open-ended subject, a very bright supervisor and Poole, the Oxford Don. For the first time in education, the spectre of failure dawned on him. This would have a massive influence on how and why he began to accumulate inferior, worthless doctorates in the future.

He was never to return to Columbia, excusing his absence on chronic illness, but intermittently kept in contact with Dunning. Finally in May 1895 he finished his thesis under the auspices of the lowly disreputable National Night University and was accepted for a PhD. JML acknowledged his thanks to Dunning for all his efforts, and had his treatise printed.[50] Without his Columbia College supervisor's and external examiners' verification, it was academically worthless. His National Night University PhD was utilised to give himself academic esteem until that hapless day some 40 years later in the House of Lords select committee when Sir William Jowitt, counsel for the British Medical Association, demonstrated JML's duplicity.

We know that in the autumn of 1895 JML's health deteriorated as his chronic symptoms returned, which gave him the excuse to write to Dunning at Columbia, informing him of this and his need to convalesce. That period of his life is not well documented, apart from his appointment as president of Amity College, College Springs, Iowa in November 1894.

From his return to America and his acceptance as president of Amity, Martin Collins describes him spending time in a Pittsburgh hospital for some months, before convalescing in an assortment of sanatoria, in

Waukesha, Wisconsin; Waco, Texas; and Denver, Colorado.[51] [52]Whilst in Waukesha, his brother James was doing some postgraduate training at the University of Chicago, a new establishment founded and funded by John D Rockefeller in 1891. Although its medical school was not founded for another seven years, JML could have utilised the faculties of the physical and biological sciences for research purposes. (Waukesha is a comparatively easy rail journey of an hour and half to the centre of Chicago). JML set out in his Curriculum Vitae (1895) that in 1893 he became a postgraduate student in Theology at the "National Night University", which was basically an evening school founded two years earlier and solely owned by its dean. It comprised of a number of so-called faculties including arts, law and presumably theology. It also included a number of health courses including dentistry, pharmacy and intriguingly, homeopathic medicine, although the word homeopathic was subsequently dropped from its title.[53] The whole establishment was closed in 1909. Be that as it may, he was awarded a dubious doctorate in Divinity (DD), on the basis of his dissertation, "The Christian Sabbatism (1894) "[54], a rehash of his Bachelor of Divinity thesis on "The Sabbatism of *Hebrews IV 9* (1891) at Glasgow University, winning the Henderson prize in Theology.

This appeared as some compensation for ceasing his PhD. Furthermore, he also stated that while residing at Providence sanatorium he met a Dr Lowber of the AdRanx Christian University of Waco, Texas (now TCU) who awarded him an honorary Doctor of Law (DLL) for services for peripatetic lecturing around Christian Universities.[55] However, it is more likely that he bought the DLL to give him a triple crown of doctorates to complete the complement of bachelor degrees from Glasgow University. Why did this academically gifted man start to accumulate such pitiful degrees?

JML had suffered two major setbacks in his professional life: firstly the incident at Creevagh when he was immeasurably out of his depth dealing with a down to earth congregation who had little respect for ethereal considerations; and secondly, his underestimation of his PhD thesis and the sheer logistics of gathering information for it from a distant European continent. This impending setback contributed to his relapse in health. Moreover, he was tempted to promote his Bachelor of Divinity dissertation for his National Night University doctorate. Indeed, his Doctor of Law from Dr Lowber was, JML concluded, acceptable to add to his other academic awards. Furthermore, he prepared his incomplete thesis, *The Political Theory of School Men and Grotius,* in May 1895 and submitted it for examination.[56]

He was perhaps too compromised to send it to Professor Dunning at Columbia for a viva voce exam and an inevitable deferral or outright rejection, so he directed it to that dubious institution, the National Night University in Chicago. After paying a suitable fee, the higher degree of PhD was conferred upon him. (Few might quibble about these trivial awards in Chicago but a different light would be cast by those Ivy League establishments on the East Coast. However, this was not the last time that JML revisited the National Night University.) Consequently he was appointed president of Amity College, College Springs, Iowa, and took up his post in November 1894.

Back in 1854 or 1855, some clergy appropriated 'unentered' indigenous native territory land, for the purpose of founding a Christian school. Advantageously it had a pure water supply from a local spring. On this site Amity College was built, being responsible for educating young people in literary, arts and scientific courses,[57] its location being a few miles from the Missouri state border.

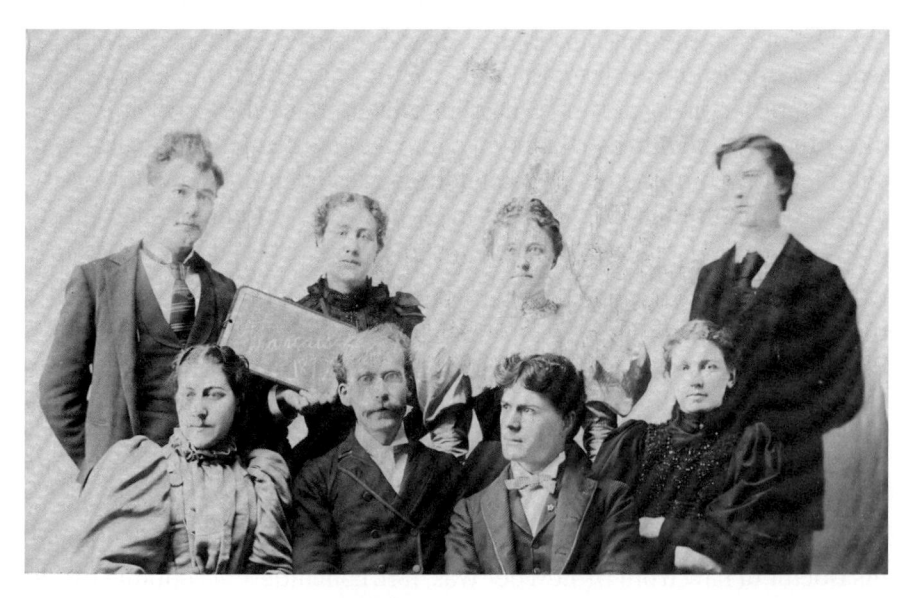

JML at Amity College

JML, an adult professional student, was transformed into being one of the youngest US college presidents around. Meanwhile, the following year his brother James was appointed its vice-president and professor of Philosophy and Civics.[58] In the meantime, their parents had settled in the community and younger brother David was connected with the college too, supposedly gaining a PhB from Amity.[59]

By the end of 1896, JML's chronic throat condition returned and in the following year he left Amity. His resignation was reluctantly accepted by the College Board who acknowledged their debt of gratitude under his stewardship.[60] There is little documentary evidence from that time. The trail seems to lead to his attendance at Dunham Homeopathic Medical School Chicago from March 1897 until August 1898, but this cannot be authenticated.[61]

He did indeed mean to train in medicine, not at this stage at Dunham, but at his old stomping ground, the National Night University, at its National Medical College or University, (its name rather fluctuates, depending on the source). From its inception in 1891 until its closure in 1909, the National Medical College's licence to train medical students had been revoked twice and had been described by the Illinois State Board of Health as "not in good standing", and in its opinion, "the worst medical school in the State of Illinois."[62] One suspects that JML would not have mentioned his attendance at this institution because some of its staff and students transferred to Dunham just before the start of the academic year (1900-1). Therefore, he was correct in saying during the select committee of the House of Lords Osteopaths Bill (1935) that he studied at Dunham, but certainly not in 1897-8.

Dunham had been set up by some dissenting staff of Hering Homeopathic Medical School Chicago, in order to revert to Hahnemann's original concepts, a kind of Classical Homeopathy, in August 1985. A building under the responsibility of Elwyn D Seaton was constructed by November that year at 370 South Wood Street, Chicago; lectures were held on site from that time onwards. In early 1900, James Tyler Kent and Harvey Harrington, both from the Postgraduate School of Homeopathics at Philadelphia, were appointed Dean and professor of Materia Medica at Dunham respectively. Interestingly, at the start of the academic year (1900-1), as previously stated, a number of staff and students from the National Medical College transferred to Dunham. This gives us a clue to JML's inclusion as a student of Dunham on the postgraduate homeopathic medical course and his graduation from Dunham in 1902, the very year it was absorbed into Hering.[63] If he had not attended the National Medical College, he would not have joined the Dunham course. It was his former connections with the National Night University that made him aware of its medical college in 1897-8 and thus enabled his transfer directly to Dunham.

In summary of his early adult years we can therefore confirm the three major themes: his undoubted academic prowess but disappointing failure as a Presbyterian minister in Ireland: his thirst for knowledge and desire to study without a decisive career focus: and his inability to convert his research into a subsequent thesis of acceptable level, being much hampered by his inability to keep to the specific matter, a consequence that seems to dog his writings throughout his life.

J Martin was not the first person found wanting by an open-ended thesis in such a distinguished faculty as Columbia, but it is a motive for his accumulation of fourth rate, trivial or worthless, doctoral awards (doctor of law DLL AdRanx, Divinity DD and PhD Night University as a result. He wasn't the only member of his family to be tempted, since both James and David utilised fellowship awards that could be gained by becoming paid members.[64] Moreover, David's use of PhD and even having a verified medical degree has never been found.[65] [66]

---

1   *Osteopathy a Basic Science* John Martin Littlejohn Memorial Lecture 1956 pp.3-5
2   National Osteopathic Archive (NOA) scanned material. J Martin Littlejohn relatives and sundry matters. Family tree. Leaf from the family bible. p.1
3   Duncan CJ, Duncan SR, Scott S. *The dynamics of scarlet fever epidemics in England and Wales in the 19th century.* Epidemiological infections 1996 Dec; 117(3): 493-9.
4   Knox WW, *A History of the Scottish People: Health in Scotland 1840-1940* Scran 2012 Chapter 3 p.3
5   So-called English Civil War was in three stages: first (1642-46); second (1648-49) both supported King Charles I against the Long parliament; and the third (1649-51) supported Charles II against the Rump parliament.
6   Wikipedia Reformed Presbyterian Church of Scotland.
7   Campbell C. *Manuscript of the Life and Times of J Martin Littlejohn* unnumbered pages
8   ibid unnumbered page.
9   According to records, Easdale Primary School on Seil Island was founded in 1877 but it may have existed in a vestigial state prior to this date.
10 Littlejohn JM NOA. Scanned material. J M Littlejohn Further Documents. *The Political Theory of School Men and Grotius* pp. 2-3.
11 "Parades and Marches - Chronology 2: Historical Dates and Events" (http://cain.ulst.ac.uk/issues/parade/chpa2.htm) . *Conflict Archive on the Internet (CAIN).* http://cain.ulst.ac.uk/issues/parade/chpa2.htm. Retrieved 28 January 2010.

12 NOA Scanned material. J M Littlejohn. Further Documents. Verified degrees and awards
13 Campbell C.
14 Rootsweb: Scotch-Irish-L The Covenanters in Ballyclabber Reformed Presby Congregation part ii
15 Littlejohn JM NOA. Scanned material. *The Political Theory of School Men and Grotius* pp. 2-3.
16 Ibid pp.2-3. Whether they continued to attend the Glasgow Seminary in 1886 is debatable as they both transferred to RPC seminary, Belfast, NI in 1885.
17 Campbell C *Manuscript:* JML Seventh in Junior Division of Logic and Rhetoric 1882/3; Fourth in Junior Class of Oriental Languages and second in examination vocabulary, Oriental languages and literature. 1883/4 unnumbered page
18 Reformed Presbyterian Church of Ireland. Website: RPC Theological Hall general information. p.1. Ian Paisley had been a student for one year.
19 Campbell C.
20 Minutes of the Southern Presbytery around June1886 p.1
21 Gregg AC incumbent minister, Cleevagh RPC *correspondence* 2011
22 Minutes of the Southern Presbytery around 7 February 1887 p.1
23 *The Covenanters in Ireland, A history of the Congregations,* Cameron Press 2010
24 Minutes of the Southern Presbytery June 1986 p.1
25 NOA, Scanned material. JM Littlejohn further documents. Verified degrees and awards.
26 Minutes of the Southern Presbytery 2 August 1887 p.1
27 Chicago College of Osteopathic Medicine archive: Biography of the Littlejohn family p.2
28 Minutes of the Southern Presbytery 7 February 1888 p.1
29 ibid 6 March 1888 pp.1-2
30 ibid 1 May 1888 p.2
31 Ibid 30 May 1888 pp.2-3
32 ibid 6 November 1888 p.3
33 Campbell, C. J M Littlejohn, Early life. 4th NOA History Society Symposium*: J Martin Littlejohn* DVD 19th June 2011
34 Chicago College of Osteopathic Medicine archive: Biography of the Littlejohn family p.2
35 Report from the Select Committee of the House of Lords: *Registration and Regulation of Osteopaths Bill [H.L.]* HMSO 1935. 3305-3308.
36 Collins M. *Osteopathy in Britain: The First hundred years* Booksurge 2005 p.37
37 Morrell MacKenzie Wikipedia Chisholm, Hugh, ed (1911). *Encyclopædia Britannica* (11th ed.). Cambridge University Press.
38 Report from the Select Committee of the House of Lords: 3320 and 3497.
39 NOA Scanned material. *The Political Theory of Schoolmen..* pp. 2-3.
40 House of Lords Select Committee, *Registration and Regulation of Osteopaths Bill*. London: HMSO, 1935 pp.227. (3415)
41 Ibid pp.2-3
42 History, Columbia University of New York. p.1 (www.columbia.edu/content/history.html.)
43 NOA Scanned material. J M Littlejohn further documents. *The Political Theory of Schoolmen..* p. 3.
44 MacCormick N. On "Public Law and the Law of Nature and Nations": A Tercentenary Lecture in the University of Edinburgh. 2007.
45 en. Wikipedia.org/wiki/Reginald_Lane_Poole.p.1
46 ibid Hugo_Grotius. p.1
47 Free Online dictionary, thesaurus and encyclopedia. p.1
48 en. Wikipedia.org/wiki/William_Archibald_Dunning p.1
49 NOA Scanned material. *The Political Theory of Schoolmen..* p. 3.
50 Ibid p.3

51 Collins M p.39
52 Report from the Select Committee of the House of Lords: 3491
53 Flexner A. *Medical Education in the United States and Canada: A Report to the Carnegie Foundation for the Advancement of Teaching.* The Carnegie Foundation.1910. pp. 212-3
54 NOA scanned material. *The Political Theory of Schoolmen..* p. 3.
55 Report from the Select Committee of the House of Lords: 3261-3266; 3393-4
56 On the front of his thesis he posts an array of academic awards: A.M., J.U.B., S.T.B., F.N.U., F.C.C.. (the first three are straight forward USA equivalents- Master of arts, Bachelor of Law and Divinity, respectively. The other two correspond to Fellows of National University and Columbia College, which are not awards.)
57 ibid 3520-1.
58 The Annals of the American Academy of Political and Social Science September 1896 vol.8 no.2 138-156
59 Gevitz N. *The DO's: Osteopathic Medicine in America* The John Hopkins University Press 1982 p. 29.
60 Collins M. pp.37-38
61 Report from the Select Committee of the House of Lords: 3497-3502.
62 Flexner A. pp.212-3
63 NOA. Scanned material. Further J M Littlejohn further documents. Waring G.P. *History of Dunham Medical School.* Edited by W H King *The History of Homeopathy and Its Institutions in America* . The Lewis Publishing Co. New York and Chicago. 1905 Volume III. Chapter 3. pp.1-9.
64 *First Announcement of announcement of the American College of Osteopathic Medicine & Surgery 1900-01* Faculty CCOM archive. F.S.Sc. (London) post fix was a dubious "club" with no permanent location.
65 Campbell E A letter to Ken Morgan, CCOM, CCOM archives 8 October 1993 p.1
66 Grigg, E R N, *Peripatetic Pioneer: William Smith MD DO (1862-1912)* Journal of the History of Medicine April 1967 p.173
"David Littlejohn graduated from the Central Medical College in St Joseph's, Missouri, November 1898- a diploma mill."

Chapter 2

The Kirksville Years (1898-1890)

In 1897, following a relapse of his throat complaint, J Martin made specific visits to consult the famous founder of osteopathy, Andrew T Still, in Kirksville, Missouri, in the earnest hope of alleviating his condition.[1] It appears that his haemorrhagic condition not only benefited from Still's ministrations, but also led JML to change direction from the National Medical College in Chicago and enter Still's medical school, the American School of Osteopathy (ASO). Initially, there must have been much mutual respect, with A T Still having the therapeutic skills to improve JML's apparent condition, and JML's credentials as the academic head of Amity College in neighbouring Iowa.

Before we explore JML's commitment to osteopathy and his time at Kirksville, we have to determine some of the principal problems that beset osteopathic evolution during those early years.

We know that A T Still started the ASO in 1892. Moreover, the first cohort of students contained a number of his own children, some children of his trusted friends, and some admirers of his skills. Without the undoubted efforts of Bill Smith, (Edinburgh medically trained), the ASO would never have prospered. In a sense, Bill was a co-founder, providing cover as lecturer in anatomy, but much more so, interpreting Still's flowery language into more conducive, scientific explanations. Moreover, osteopathy emerged from magnetic healing, principally by changing individual mental attitudes, and, allied with bone setting skills, became a practical physical craft successfully employed throughout America and Europe. However, these two ingredients did not dove-tail quite succinctly as has been suggested by other commentators.

No doubt the simple bone-out-of-place analogy was easy for patients and students to understand. Additionally, A T Still's down to earth explanations to many of his patients may have portrayed their sufferings as physically based, although many might have assumed and partly ascribed them religiously as expiation for past misdemeanours or sinfulness in their individual lives. Still's ability to formulate simple physical reasons for pain underpinned much more complex problems of spiritual, emotional, mental and practical sociological considerations which could be addressed through magnetic healing. Although Still understood these different ideas he was unable to explain to Bill Smith or others the true nature of his therapy, or for them to quite understand it either, (not helped by Still's apparent grudging explanation of his magnetic healing origins). Moreover, his failure to admit his previous involvement in magnetic healing to pursue a bonesetting ethos, based on a physical diagnosis and treatment, fitted his situation well. By specifically concentrating on simple vertebral displacements that could influence these distressing complaints, by manipulative realignment, he found a successful formula for eliminating distress and disability.

A T Still had first hand practical experience not only of new settlers passing through Kansas on their way to California and Oregon, but also those individuals in homesteads and farms spread throughout Kansas, Missouri and Iowa in isolated and scattered communities. The former with fears and expectations as they journeyed through sometimes hostile and rugged terrain before reaching their intended destination, and the latter with ambitions of raising cattle and sheep and tilling virgin land for crops amidst the vagaries of pestilence and weather. It was among these groups that AT Still perfected his clinical skills. He was able to address more important psychological, emotional, sociological and demographic elements by using practical simplistic explanations of bones and vertebrae being out of place. His success was affirmed when he built a hospital/ clinic in Kirksville Missouri, the infirm travelled to him rather than the other way round. No longer capable of dealing with a surge in patient numbers, it became imperative to train other practitioners to his capabilities.

In 1892, the American School of Osteopathy was founded by A T Still with essential support from Bill Smith, willing to teach basic anatomy and useful to interpret Still's particular expressive language in a more scientific way. Furthermore, Smith was able to evolve Still's osteopathy beyond bone setting and magnetic healing. The ASO offered very basic medical training combined with rudimentary manipulative demonstrations. It appeared to prosper for four years, until the time when Still's family applied for state accreditation as a bona fide medical school. Bill Smith had remained at the school for a year but kept in touch with proceedings after leaving. Nevertheless, it was to Smith that the Still family turned after failing to gain state accreditation for the school. Accordingly, Smith successfully steered the ASO through to state approval, the outcome of which defined osteopathy's further development and direction.

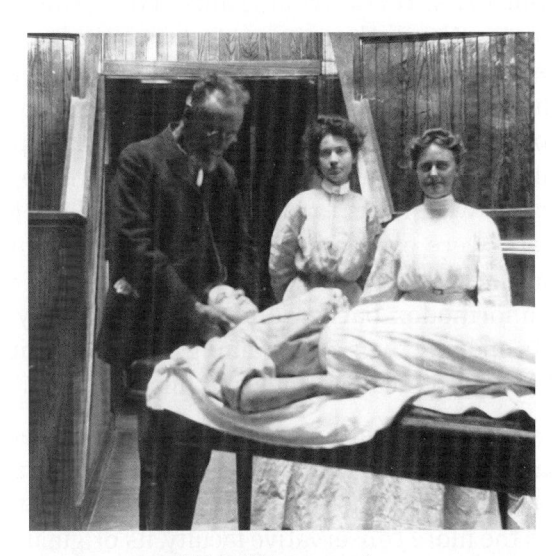

A T Still in practice

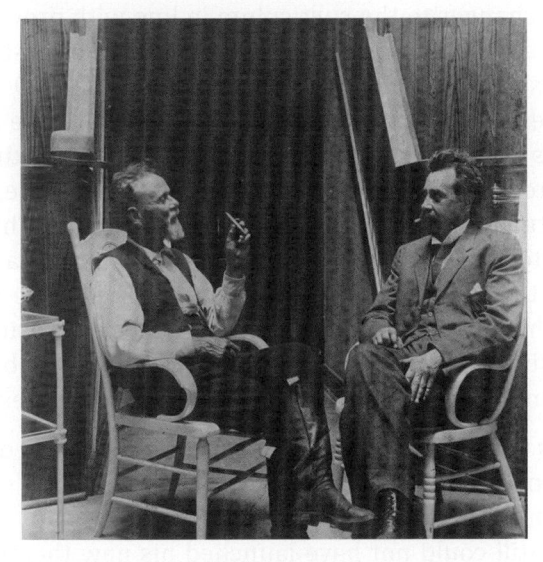

A T Still and Bill Smith in discussion

In 1896-7, a large student intake, aided and abetted by state accreditation, whilst at the same time adopting such necessary curricular changes as was demanded by the Missouri state legislature, added to A T Still's general discomfort and disapproval. Moreover, he somehow sensed that their introduction to this revised course did not translate into an effective osteopathic training. Nor did he gain comfort from the impersonal nature of having to deal with so many students. Although his children seemed delighted with the influx of such numbers and the resultant financial rewards, the loss of curriculum control and family atmosphere weighed heavily on Still. His frustration became even more apparent by the increase in faculty, which was to include the three Littlejohn brothers, who, with others, were expressly responsible for updating the course to include more medical sciences. Still could have been more open in admitting his unorthodox background but he was very conscious of former students opening their own training establishments on his ideas and reaping the rewards academically and financially.

More importantly, he felt that his school was rapidly metamorphosing away from magnetic healing with bonesetting, into an alien criterion based around medical subjects. This not only continued to trouble him but also divided the more conservative faculty, its original graduates and many students. Bill Smith and the Littlejohn brothers had been recruited to implement changes to the curriculum in line with provisions of state accreditation as expressed by Lou Stephens, Missouri state governor. Moreover, this new governor no longer vetoed the ASO state charter, as his predecessor had done. In 1896, he conferred state accreditation to the ASO as a bona fide medical school, thereby setting it along a tortuous route, dependent upon its survival, of course, towards its ultimate destination within conventional medicine. This event has been highlighted in the annals of osteopathic history as a great victory but, perhaps, this epoch requires further scrutiny before reaching that conclusion. This pivotal struggle between traditional osteopathic core curricula versus orthodox medical subjects continued to be the focus of attention for many decades, perhaps even to present times.

Crucial to this was Bill Smith's central role in those early days, teaching anatomy, acting as a sounding board for much of Still's notions and interpreting his ideas in a more conventional way. Without his intervention, Still could not have launched his new therapy to a wider public, and his training establishment to fresh recruits, willing to enter a state accredited medical school amidst various critical comments from orthodox medicine, without Smith's guidance.[2] Although the school managed to train three modest cohorts of osteopaths, it was Smith's pursuit of a state charter as a medical school that, if it was to succeed, became an irreversible contradiction in terms of its curricula, character and rationale. Furthermore, this particular crisis was exacerbated by those that pushed for further advances and reforms in so-called osteopathic subjects rather than medical ones, necessitating a genuine desire to explain how osteopathy might work, and its effectiveness. From this we can conclude that early practitioners were open to different ideas but were never able to stray too far from Still's vigilant gaze.

Without a state charter, the ASO would probably have failed. Bill Smith's involvement in its eventual ratification was paramount. Whereas Chiropractic relied on B J Palmer's, its founder's son, considerable publicity acumen and entrepreneurial skills to boost student entry, there appeared to be no osteopathic equivalent. Bill Smith's contribution was to embrace all orthodox medical school subjects, except materia medica, according to the Missouri state diktats, into the ASO curriculum. It was to be spread over four terms of five months duration each term.[3] A decade further on, Flexner, in his report on North American medical schools, extols the merits of high school education of four years in the state of Missouri that, on matriculation, can lead to entry into the esteemed state university. Moreover, he abhors the fact that no Missouri chartered medical school demands similar qualifications for entry and yet does not question the most rudimentary of schooling standards for their own student admission. Consequently, the Missouri medical schools were overcrowded with inadequate students, and poorly trained to boot.

Furthermore, Flexner was dismayed at the quality of these Missouri institutions and their graduates compared with other states, describing them as 'some of the poorest in the country'.[4] Nevertheless, the ASO charter led to a three-fold increase in graduates in 1898, a further increase the following year and nearly seven times that number in the 1899 cohort.[5] Consequently, this post-charter surge, from 1899 onwards, led to an enlarged ASO faculty to facilitate training.

C M T Hulett was appointed as Dean in 1898 or 1899 to oversee the ASO's expansion, but his tenure was not long.[6]

Controlling such a dramatic surge in entrants and supervising their training required experience and talent. No wonder the process threw up a multitude of problems. A T Still must have been taken aback by the scale of demand for places. From being a small personal school where everyone was part of a large extended family, it developed into an amorphous institution of nameless faces. Consequently, A T Still called on his sons, Harry and, especially, Charlie, to bear most of the responsibilities and workload. The award of a state charter had reinvigorated the ASO but at a price, and more importantly, as stated previously, had filled the curricula with medical subjects as opposed to osteopathic.

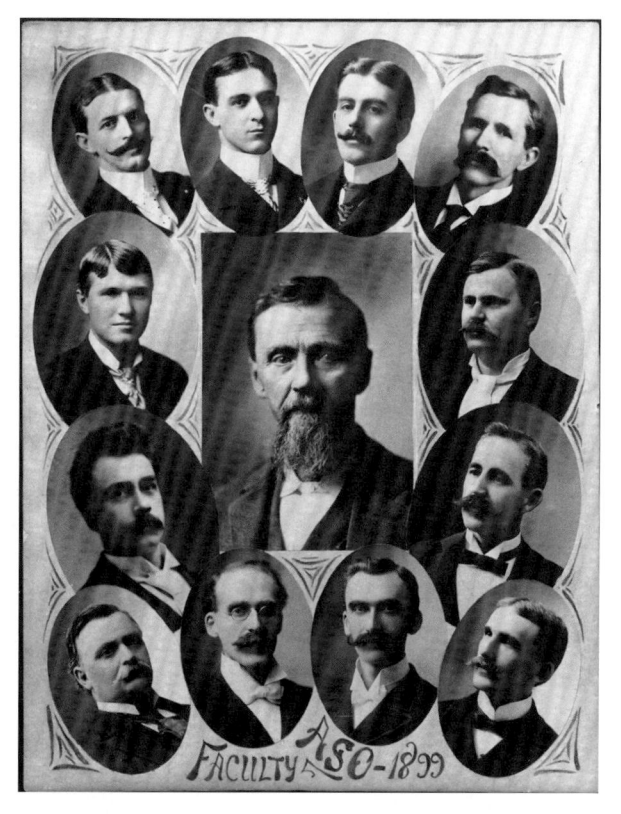

ASO faculty 1899

In the past, Harry, twin brother of Herman, had been the first family member A T Still taught to help him during his peripatetic times as a 'lightning bone setter'.[7] His children Harry, Herman, Charlie, Blanche and beloved Fred, all graduated from the first class of students at the ASO in 1893. The following year Harry moved away from Kirksville to Chicago in order to set up an osteopathic practice. Indeed, he was successful in doing this and then selling it on. He used the same formula several times to open thriving clinics in St. Louis and New York. Moreover, he was very perceptive in picking those he could trust, family friends from ASO graduates: Charles Hazzard, Carl McConnell and Arthur Hildreth were appointed to assist in Chicago.[8] When AT Still summoned Harry back to help run the school, it was to these trusted colleagues he turned to join the faculty. These allies became Harry's ears and eyes within the enlarged faculty. Additionally, they were joined by Dr C W Proctor PhD, author of two books published during his time at Kirksville, *Brief Course in General Chemistry* and *Brief Course in Physiological Chemistry*, and by the three Littlejohn brothers, J Martin (JML), James and David, at different stages.[9]

The Littlejohn brothers took up their respective ASO faculty appointments at different times. JML said it was in February 1898 [10] and on another occasion, September of that year.[11] He entered the ASO as its professor of Physiology. James joined in the spring term as professor of Surgery, Histology and Pathology,[12] followed by David in September 1888 as professor of Chemistry, Urinalysis and Public Health.[13]

During his interrogation at the House of Lords Select Committee, Sir William Jowitt KC, counsel for the British Medical Association, presses JML further on his time as the ASO professor of physiology. JML says his time was taken up with physiological experimentation. However there is no indication that any took place during this time. Moreover, Jowitt finds it inconceivable for a person without qualifications in the field of physiology could be appointed so.[14] Jowitt's assumption was based on the rigid professorial system imposed on British academia, compared with an easier, laissez-faire transatlantic interpretation of US professor entitlement.

JML had completed an undergraduate course in physiology during the academic year (1897-8) at the National Medical School, Chicago under the auspices of its National Night University. Furthermore, JML cites his attendance at Anderson's Medical School, Glasgow, as evidence of his ability to teach physiology.[15] Although there is no record of his official attendance, brother James qualified there in 1892, so it is possible that JML could have been present at some of these lectures and borrowed textbooks and lecture notes under James's forbearance. Additionally, while at Amity College (1884-1887), JML's lessons might have included science (James's role as his deputy might have overlapped). Among the most popular books for teachers of elementary physiology, one was written by the celebrated Thomas Huxley. This was a descriptive, erudite explanation of the workings of the human body in balanced function. Far from being elementary, it was just the basis on which to demonstrate to ASO students with no comprehension of the subject how osteopathic principles and practice can be illustrated physiologically. Huxley constructed his book to appeal to the highest common factor among his readers. This would have appealed to JML too.[16] Moreover, Huxley was an autodidact and a descriptive anatomist, his writing style was clear and would certainly have found favour among early osteopathic pioneers, although his ruthless logic and scientific credence would have been dismissive of osteopathy's views. Be that as it may, there is evidence that JML was familiar with the subject and capable of teaching basic physiology to his brief.

Whatever his qualifications, he entered the ASO as its professor of Physiology.[17]

In a sense, the brothers' arrival at Kirksville was proportionate to their desire to commit to the osteopathic profession. Having undertaken some medical training at Central Michigan Medical College, St Joseph, Michigan, David remained within the profession for two decades, before branching out independently as a medical officer in Public Health.[18] James developed into a highly regarded lecturer and was in the vanguard of osteopathic restructuring towards orthodox medicine. JML must have been the catalyst for his brothers' entry, initially extolling the virtues of his osteopathic treatment from the master himself, AT Still.

In the past JML would relapse into his debilitating illness at eventful times, usually during crisis periods, strongly suggesting emotional factors to his complaint. This type of condition was grist to the mill for A T Still, and accordingly JML's symptoms improved under his attention. Many perceived Still as an alternative medical Abraham Lincoln, perhaps some of his eminence acted as a compass for JML to follow.[19] He had found his safe harbour, no longer was JML distracted by extraneous enthusiasms and restlessness to pursue other causes. This odyssey had had many twists and turns before he reached Osteopathy. Still's "new healing" lifted his spirit, instilling (pun intended) buoyancy and commitment which would continue, through thick and thin, further trials and tribulations, for the rest of his life. Nonetheless, his esteem for A T Still and family and those faculty members allied to the Stills would oscillate dramatically too.

Chapter 2

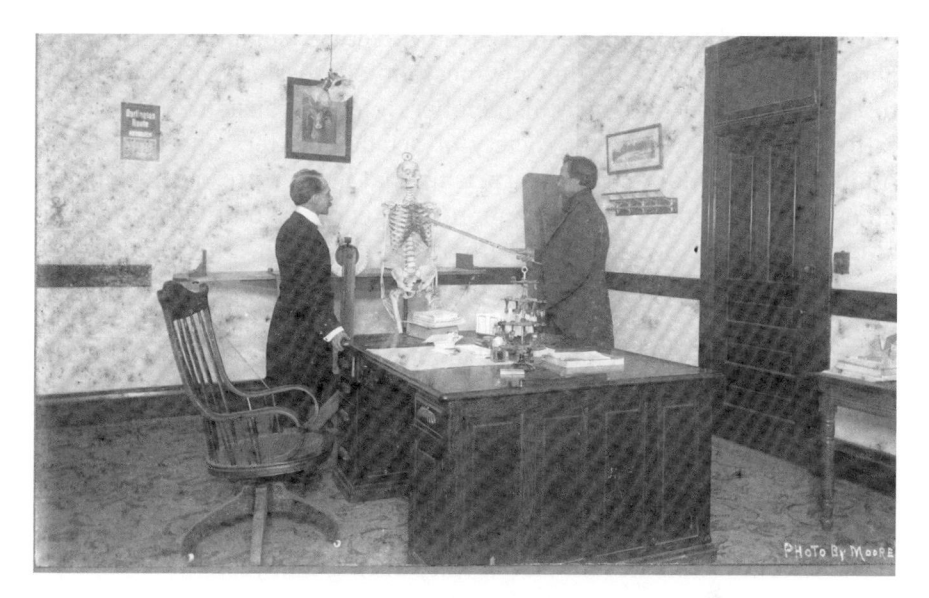

A T Still and JML

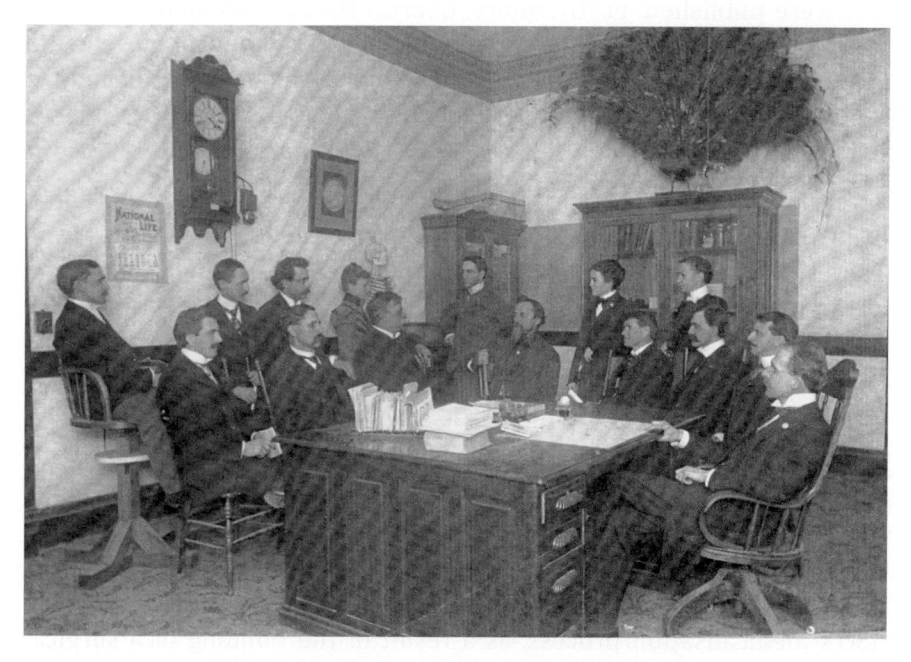

JML in the Chair with the Kirksville faculty

Previously in July 1898, he had given a lecture, somewhat ethereally entitled, "Osteopathy in line of apostolic succession with Medicine" to the assembled audience of members of the transient, peripatetic, rather grandiosely named, Society of Science, Letters and Art, at the Addison Hall, London. It was surprising that he was presenting a paper on osteopathy after a bare four months attendance on the ASO faculty, although he had been A T Still's patient for much longer. JML must have discussed its rationale with him and perhaps, his fellow Scot, Bill Smith, on a number of occasions. It is to JML's credit that he understood, more or less, what both had revealed and, importantly, how osteopathy could evolve further. Indeed, those present in Addison Hall were so suitably enthralled that they awarded him a Gold Medal and eligibility of membership of the Society that accorded him a fellowship and the suffix, FSSA (London). Consequently, he was invited back the following year.[20] No doubt it was his zest for osteopathy that had persuaded James and David to follow him into the ASO faculty during that year.

Meanwhile, an infectious spirit of innovation and evolution of osteopathy came forth as a crop of osteopathic textbooks by Bill Smith, Charles Hazzard, Carl McConnell, C W Proctor and two volumes of physiology by JML were published. Furthermore, Charles Hazzard studied Per Ling's gymnastic passive and active techniques, whose rhythmical movements could well have been the forerunner of osteopathic articulatory technique. Hence, The 'bone out of place' lesion had another characteristic - that of reduced mobility.

Furthermore, Hazzard and JML collaborated on notions of nerve disturbances directly affecting and influencing the function of an organ. They suggested the proposition of "inhibition and stimulation" along an "irritable nerve" could be manipulated through physical pressure from its vasomotor centre. In addition, JML worked closely with Carl McConnell and his brothers too, proposing that spinal lesions attributed to a weakening of the immune system, thereby making an individual more prone to illness, whilst reducing or eliminating vertebral lesions boosted the body's ability to fight off disease.[21] At some stage, the Scottish quartet of Bill Smith and the Littlejohns started to irritate not only Arthur Hildreth but also A T Still himself.

It all culminated in a series of unfortunate incidents increasing the ASO's medicalisation process, as a result of the building of a surgical sanatorium, probably built at the behest of James Littlejohn, professor of major surgery. It is difficult to understand why the establishment of a post-operative building would create such an outburst of wrath, but it did, with A T Still again railing against an osteopathic drift towards medicine, "*My school was chartered to teach osteopathy only*".[22] He took a dim view of expanding his classical interpretation of osteopathy to embrace further medical disciplines such as surgery, but the die was cast.[23] In hindsight, once the decision was taken to pursue state charter for his beloved ASO, there were only two outcomes, survive as a proper medical school with a constant stream of enthusiastic student entrants, or return to its unaccredited status with a dramatic drop in student numbers. Besides, the Still family benefitted greatly in the financial security offered by the ASO's expansion. It certainly suited the family to put the blame on the Littlejohns for the post-operative sanatorium, a culmination for converting the school to an acceptable Missouri medical college irrespective of its vestigial nature. Although A T Still had considerable reservations about allowing Bill Smith to guide the ASO towards greater medical curricular input, he left implementation to Smith and the Littlejohns. The family appeared to allow their father's wrath to build, whilst offering the support for Smith and the Littlejohns to pursue reforms and, more importantly, funds to continue to fill the coffers.

In fact, there was a ground swell countermovement among some students and faculty, approved by the founder, to resist not only further adaptation of the curriculum but propose a return to a purer golden age of his "lightning bone setting" based on magnetic healing. Whether this was romantic posturing to publicly rebuke such orthodox reforms but privately enjoy undoubted considerable financial rewards, we will never know, but it suited Still's family and allies to take such a stand. JML knew that Dunham Homeopathic Medical School in Chicago had been founded by dissident Hering Homeopathic Medical school staff for precisely the same reason, to pursue essential Hahnemann doctrines.[24] At some stage JML was not only the ASO Professor of Physiology but following C M T Hulett's resignation as the ASO Dean, he was also appointed to that office. Meanwhile, Hildreth had started a practice in St Louis with Harry Still.

At such time Charlie Still, and to a lesser extent Harry, ran the ASO affairs for their father who took a back seat, but who was always ready to rant against medical subjects being taught, bravura that many students might have gleefully supported. Meanwhile, Charlie Still appeared as quite a diplomat, keeping all members of the faculty to all intents and purposes reasonably equable. Notably during 1899, Charlie Still, his wife, and daughter Gladys, attended David Littlejohn's marriage to Mary Forbes, sister of Bill Smith's wife, at a small wedding ceremony with father, James Littlejohn and JML co-officiating. Also Blanche Still, Charles' sister, was present, who according to some sources, was being wooed by JML among a number of suitors.[25] At this stage, some of Still's family continued to uphold good relations with Smith and the Littlejohns. Indeed, it was during this "honeymoon" period that C M T Hulett resigned as dean, to be replaced by JML. Hulett might well have been finding the position too exacting: trying to integrate an intake of nearly 200 freshman students; coping with limited lecture room and clinic space; plus incorporating new faculty with an ever changing curriculum. JML's credentials, (his previous experience in running a much smaller Amity College,) recommended him to the Stills as the man to provide cohesion and solve innumerable difficulties. Whether this job was a poisoned chalice soon became evident with disgruntled senior staff and the Still family's earlier confidence in him and his fellow Scots disappearing very rapidly.

Bill Smith and the Littlejohns seemed wholly different to their peers, better educated, more medically orientated and, perhaps, more persuasive in discussions. They became the perfect fall-guys for Charlie and Harry Still to blame, playing off their father and his faculty allies against all curricular changes required by state charter, as represented by the Scots. What didn't help was an increasing antipathy between them and Arthur Hildreth, a devoted A T Still ally, when he joined the ASO faculty. It became a cause celebre of too much medicalisation as opposed to osteopathy, supposedly at the behest of Smith and the Littlejohns, alienating them from the remaining faculty and some students.[26]

James Littlejohn had been hired as the ASO professor of surgery. It was probably his proposal to build and equip a post-operative sanatorium commensurate with carrying out minor and major surgery. Its commissioning and construction was effected without A T Still's knowledge but clearly sanctioned by members of the Still family. A T Still was invited to open the sanatorium at its inauguration, but, clearly exasperated by the increasing ASO medicalisation, this event appears as the last straw. Later, under Hildreth, it was closed but mysteriously reopened a few years on.[27] Firstly JML was summarily dismissed from his post as Dean after five months tenure, and Hildreth was appointed by the Still family as his replacement. The incident provoked much discord among the Littlejohns, with Smith tagging along, rather reluctantly. It abruptly severed any remaining fragile co-existence within the ASO faculty in August 1899.[28] Although they had been hired on the sound grounds that they were employed to fulfil the charter's edicts, their plea was magnificent, pertinent but futile. Consequently the Scottish quartet were dismissed from the faculty, Smith instantly, the Littlejohns remaining until the end of the academic year. David left at the end of January 1900 with an ASO physician's certificate,[29] JML and James in June of that year.[30]

Arthur Hildreth had always been part of the dependable Still network, his family association went back to his boyhood when the itinerant bonesetter A T Still would visit the family homestead in those difficult peripatetic times. Hildreth became an astute politician who had sided with A T Still over opposition to the postoperative sanatorium, and this loyalty did not go unnoticed either. Meanwhile, It was in the interest of the Still family to criticise those aspects of the state charter that they opposed without admitting that the charter would not have been granted without such implementations. Indeed without it, student entry would have been paltry compared with the numbers flocking to the ASO. Perhaps Smith and the Littlejohns, especially JML (who was presumably smarting over his removal from his role as Dean), had underestimated Hildreth. Certainly JML was intellectually more persuasive, superiorly educated and had experience of participating and running faculties. But he could also be obstinate, somewhat naïve and antagonistic. On the other hand Hildreth was an effective practitioner, businessman, and resolute loyalist, determined to support and appearing to implement the cogent wishes of A T Still. Subsequently, he was to emerge as an outstanding politician to further the advance of osteopathic state legislation.[31] By raising Hildreth's appointment with Charlie Still and the ASO trustees, the Littlejohns and Smith in tow not only alienated the rest of the faulty but also much of the student body.[32]

How ironic to have been fired for the very reason that they had been hired, to implement the conditions of the state charter. Subsequently, Hildreth summarily closed the surgical sanatorium and hand picked certain osteopaths to fill those vacancies in the faculty.[33] However, Smith had probably become less enthusiastic to the cause as the matter escalated, he returned to the ASO to teach intermittently during 1904 and also 1908. He is remembered with much affection. For some time,

JML tenaciously pursued a legal vendetta with the Still family, almost to the point of obsession. All three brothers moved to Chicago to create their own osteopathic college, based on their own interpretation from a distance, without resistance or constraint from the Still family.

The feud between the Stills and Littlejohns erupted over the building of the surgical sanatorium, but its origins stem from Governor Stephens awarding the ASO with the Missouri state charter. By committing his school to such a radical alteration, A T Still could not reconstitute its modus vivendi based on bone setting and magnetic healing, however hard he tried to do so. Nor could he have envisaged that each new intake would dwarf the earliest three small student cohorts. The charter brought great numbers of students with increased entrants of those matriculating from high schools. The personal attention prescribed for early students could not be maintained in cohorts seven times that number either. In practical terms, the genie was out of the bottle, the alternative being no charter, few students and modest financial return.

Smith and the Littlejohns could never imagine those long treks A T Still made across Missouri, the settlements and townships sprouting up, some failing to prosper, and those calamitous crop catastrophes that beset homesteads. Smith and the Littlejohns had knowledge of physical ailments, epidemics and other diseases manifested among these communities, but not the emotional crises and sociological havoc that was at the heart of A.T. Still's experience. During those pioneering days, some families welcomed Still as a friend, not as an eccentric snake-oil salesman. He never forgot their kindness. Trust, as Phineas Parkhurst Quimby, the eminent magnetic healer, would say, is a principal element in a person's recovery to health, and this mutual reliance was at the heart of his itinerant practice. Certainly JML had been struck by Still's methods as one of his admiring patients. His ability to address JML with simple explanations of his complicated chronic ill health and then treat it successfully caused him to convert to osteopathy. Quimby would have explained to JML, it was not education he required but re-education.[34] Central to Still's osteopathy was the use of physical treatment to aid most illnesses based on his sociological, emotional and psychological experiential knowledge. It was unfortunate that the bone out of place was given so much emphasis and that Quimby's insights were not furthered.

This conflict of retaining those core subjects based around Still's traditional methods not only continued to divide an emerging profession but also fuel personal attacks on those who pushed for further advances and reforms. It exacerbated a genuine desire to explain how osteopathy worked within its clinical effectiveness in a general and more specific way.

Broadly, too much emphasis was placed on the osteopathic lesion, 'bone out of place', being responsible for all kinds of debilities. Gradually group vertebral lesions were mentioned, causing areas of poor mobility. Consequently, the lesion was responsible for impaired mobility within one spinal segment or among a group of vertebrae. A few osteopaths investigated Per Ling's ideas on health based on physical intervention through active and passive movements but not as thoroughly as one would have wished. There were other medical sources at the time making connection between health and physical intervention that demanded further study too. However, A T Still did not approve of too much investigation by others. Any person questioning the validity or existence of such a lesion, which was largely built on observation and palpatory skill, was quite likely to be lambasted with needless personal attacks rather than healthy debate. Evidently, heated discussions over attempts to modify, adapt and refine osteopathic theory and practice inevitably deteriorated into personal diatribe among those who respected A T Still's wishes and those prepared to challenge his authoritative edicts. There was always rhetoric to defend what was, in reality, unsubstantiated dogma and a yearning to return to a supposed bygone golden age that never really existed.

Perhaps JML and others did perceive A T Still as a bonesetter, pure and simple, unable to explain his methods in a cogent succinct way. Moreover, Bill Smith must have spent hours discussing his own interpretation to the Littlejohns, but even Smith was helpless in defining the true nature of Still's claim. In a sense JML's own approach to describing osteopathy leaves one as a prospector for gold:- there are a few precious particles among quite a bit of grit in the prospecting pan, picking his gold specks of knowledge remains most difficult to do but worth pursuing. Predictably Bill Smith {who had cosigned some of JML's vitriolic letters) was forgiven and he duly returned to lecture at the ASO intermittently throughout the 1900s. His contribution was paramount during those early years, ably assisted by the Littlejohns, Hazzard, McConnell, and Proctor. They furthered osteopathic evolution to a more academic and intellectual level than A T Still was ever able to achieve. However, relations between the Littlejohns and Stills reached new depths of mutual personal recrimination and denigration, which continued for some years.

---

1. Collins M. *Osteopathy in Britain: The First hundred years* Booksurge 2005 pp. 39-40.
2. Booth E R History *of Osteopathy* The Author Cincinnati Ohio 1924 pp. 447-450
3. Gevitz N. *The DO's: Osteopathic Medicine in America* The John Hopkins University Press 1982 pp. 28-9.
4. Flexner A. *Medical Education in the United States and Canada: A Report to the Carnegie Foundation for the Advancement of Teaching.* The Carnegie Foundation. 1910. pp. 258-9.
5. Gevitz N. Notes 34: "according to figures cited by E.M.Violette, the number of graduates jumped from 48 in 1897, to 136 in 1898, 185 in 1899, and 317 in 1900. See his *History of Adair County* (Kirksville: Journal Printing, 1911, p.264.") p.159.
6. Booth E R *Tribute to* p663.
7. ibid pp.17-18.
8. Hildreth A G *The Lengthening Shadow of Andrew Taylor Still* The Author 1938 pp.80-81
9. Booth E R p.285.
10. NOA scanned material. J M Littlejohn Further documents. *Littlejohns' deposition statements made in September 1900.* p.16.
11. Report from the Select Committee of the House of Lords: *Registration and Regulation of Osteopaths Bill [H.L.]* HMSO 1935. 3498-3502; 3518.
12. Gevitz N. p. 36
13. Ibid. p. 29-30.
14. Ibid 3497
15. Ibid 3519
16. Huxley, Thomas H. *Lessons in Elementary Physiology* MacMillan, London 1870 fourth edition
17. Littlejohn D. *Public Health Administration* Am J Public Health Nations Health. 1932 September; 22(9): 978–982.
18. Trowbridge C. *Andrew Taylor Still 1828-1917* Truman State University Press 1991 p. 174.
19. Booth E R. *History of Osteopathy and twentieth-century medical practice* The Caxton Press. Cincinnati 1924 pp.38-42
20. Collins M. p.11.
21. Gevitz N. pp. 29-33.
22. Trowbridge C. p.176
23. Ibid p.176.
24. Waring, GP. Chapter III Dunham Medical College OF Chicago. *History of Homeopathy and its Institutions in America;* Ed: William Harvey King Presented by Sylvain Cazalet p.3.
25. Berchtold T *To Teach, To Heal, To Serve! A History of the Chicago College of Osteopathic Medicine 1900-1975.* Chicago College of Osteopathic Medicine, 1975 p. 17.
26. Trowbridge C. p.178
27. Ibid p.178
28. Hildreth A G pp.122-124
29. *Littlejohns' deposition statements made in September 1890.* p.32.
30. ibid p.2 and pp.36-44 respectively.
31. Gevitz N. p.50.
32. Littlejohn J M *Trustees of the ASO 23rd November 1899* NOA Scanned Material J Martin Littlejohn documents
33. Trowbridge C. pp. 177-8.
34. Fuller R C *Mesmerism and the American Cure of Souls* University of Pennsylvania Press. Philadelphia. 1982. pp.129-133.

Chapter 3

The Chicago Years

We know that J Martin Littlejohn received his Diploma in Osteopathy (DO) in January 1900, and brother David was awarded his physician certificate at the same time.[1] James Littlejohn did not receive one and neither requested one especially, after being told that $200 of his salary had been withheld. If he wished to obtain a diploma then he should deposit a further $100 in addition to the $200 owed to him, and discuss the matter with Warren Hamilton, the American School of Osteopathy (ASO) secretary and school treasurer. As far as James was concerned the subject was objectionable and out of the question.[2] Furthermore, a week or so after receiving his diploma, JML resigned from the faculty as professor of physiology but continued to appeal to Warren Hamilton for unpaid salary demands.[3] It clearly took some months for the brothers to extricate themselves from Kirksville.

They had learnt valuable lessons in the pros and cons of running an osteopathic medical school and also the direction they needed to take. JML had been the ASO dean of the faculty for only five months, but even so, this time was invaluable. He had been at the heart of the organisation - especially one that maintained a small faculty to teach a large number of students. The treasurer Hamilton no doubt slept easily at night, warm in the knowledge that his staff wages were modest, while ever-increasing money, through students' and patients' fees, flowed in.[4] And the Littlejohns knew it. They were well aware of the financial gains occurring in such an establishment in a remote Midwestern town such as Kirksville. Better surely to locate such an establishment within a vibrant city like Chicago.

However, a number of other things were on JML's mind, namely his own lack of medical qualifications compared with his brother James, and a growing, romantic flickering, perhaps a need to settle down.

In the Midwest much of the commercial influence came from Chicago. There were some rumours about transferring the ASO there, literally lock, stock and barrel. Moreover, Harry Still had run a highly successful practice in Chicago. Perhaps ASO faculty members had discussed the

39

subject, especially those with experience of practicing there. Osteopaths such as Harry, Carl McConnell, and Arthur Hildreth all had real expert knowledge of Chicago as an ideal location for an osteopathic school. This chatter about locating the school to Chicago would only have confirmed the Littlejohn brothers' own considerations about having their own college in the city. James had studied there and previously too, David is thought to have had some partial medical training at Central Michigan College, St Josephs, (barely 100 miles away) in 1897. However this clashes with another author who cites David Littlejohn graduated from the Central Medical College in St Joseph's, Missouri, November 1898 - a diploma mill.[5] [6] It is more likely that he is associated with the latter due to its proximity to Amity College, his place of study in 1897 and Kirksville in 1898.

More importantly, JML had utilised his connections with the National Night University to furnish himself with doctorates of Philosophy (PhD) and Divinity (DD). Further future connection with that institution's National Medical College might provide him with a medical qualification too. (Even his eldest brother William had resigned from the Presbyterian Church as Minister to retrain as a physician. Although he steered clear of osteopathy, he worked for many years as a general practitioner in the United States.[7]) It was to this end that JML now turned his thoughts - towards fulfilling his need to complete an MD course. He returned to the familiar portals of the National Night University, in order to renew his acquaintance with its dean. But before discussing this, we must mention his pursuits of the heart.

Although JML might have cherished thoughts for A T Still's youngest daughter, the pretty Blanche, his somewhat inappropriate 21st birthday present to her was, rather than her preferred gift of flowers, a set of encyclopaedias, a quirky expression of his fondness and a measure of his permanent intent. It has been suggested that his present was not discarded, instead being utilised by her children for reference purposes in future years, very much in the way that JML would have wished.[8]

Blanche had many other admirers, and rising above them all to win her heart was George M Laughlin. They married in April 1900.[9] Not only did Laughlin defend A T Still's more traditional approach, a diplomatic deference to his father in law, but also he became one of the most influential osteopathic pioneers, championing underprivileged rural students. These hopeful recruits came from homesteads and small towns whose parents could ill afford further college costs, raw entry candidates not necessarily ideal for raising academic standards in osteopathic medical schools.[10] It was fitting that some weeks after the wedding the uninvited JML and his brothers left Kirksville for Chicago. Besides, in July 1900, brother James was to marry Edith Williams, an ASO graduate from Tennessee, who was to play an important part together with her husband in osteopathic politics and academia.[11]

Meanwhile, JML was making suitable plans to return to Britain and marry Mabel Alice Thompson of Ipswich, Suffolk. The previous year, he had celebrated the wedding of his sister, Elizabeth, known as Bessie, to Tom Anthony in Ipswich. It is thought that Mabel was one of her bridesmaids. During that family occasion, JML and Mabel became suitably enamoured with each other very quickly. It was common then, just as now, for romance to flourish among friends introduced by brothers and sisters. It has been thought that Bessie and Mabel's friendship came from their mutual attendance at a training establishment nearby. It would have been an honour for Mabel to be chosen as Bessie's bridesmaid. The courtship would have been successfully sustained by correspondence, even though distances were great, the excitement and anticipation of long-awaited letters would add to the romance. [12] JML had found his beloved Mabel.

Prior to the wedding plans he contacted his old friend, the dean of the National Night University, Chicago. The good dean informed JML that a number of his staff and most of the students of his National Medical College were transferring to Dunham Medical School for the academic year of 1900-1.[13] This arrangement coincided with Dunham affiliating with the postgraduate Homeopathics' medical school in Philadelphia. James Tyler Kent, one of its leading lights, became Dunham's dean and had been responsible for a similar postgraduate course as its sister Philadelphian school. It was a two-year course leading to an award of an MD (Dunham).

This situation ideally suited JML: he could assist his brothers in establishing their own osteopathic school while at the same time gain his MD. He appears to have entered the postgraduate course by firstly attending the National Medical College course (in 1897-8) and secondly by misrepresenting his Night University awarded PhD and a rather dubious 'FRS' to affirm his academic credence. It appears JML dropped the 'L' from the tenuous 'FRSL' originally picked up in London by paying a fee to become a member of the Royal Society of Literature.[14] This fellowship was usually awarded to a celebrated literary writer and one cannot envisage JML in such a position. However, the use of "FRS", Fellow of the Royal Society being indeed an august honour, conveys a fellowship of even greater standing.[15] This suggests Charlie Still's accusation that JML's claim to have lectured on 19th July 1899 to the Royal Society of Science at Crystal Palace, London, was bogus, was right.[16] Furthermore it added more vitriol to the vendetta between the two families.

Dunham Medical School's own existence arose from homeopathic differences.

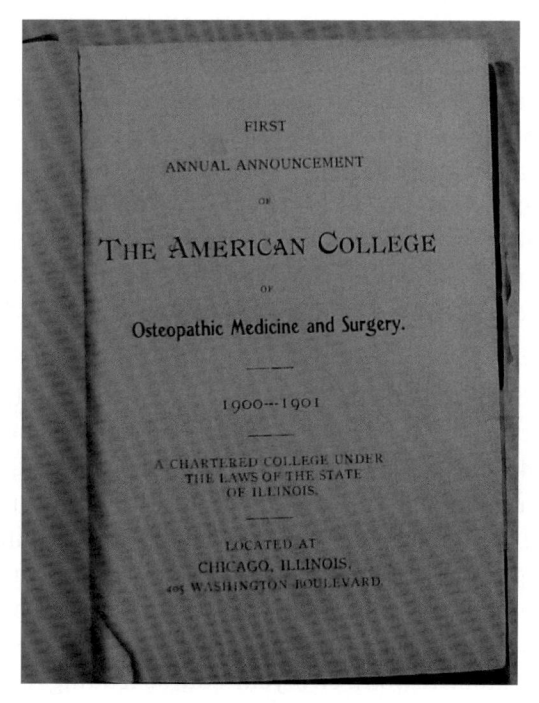

The first ACOMS prospectus

It had been founded in 1895 by dissident staff from Hering Medical College. Its ethos was to train students based on Hahnemann's original precepts, described as "pure Homeopathy" and, of course, the usual 'personal difficulties arising in the faculty of Hering Medical School'.[17] After JML's experiences at the ASO Kirksville, he well understood the intricacies and petty notions circulating within college walls. By 1902,

Dunham authorities awarded JML his MD, duly recognising him among the ten most eminent members of its alumni.[18] At the same time, negotiations with Hering medical school were well advanced enough for Dunham to be assimilated within its older sister college, all differences having been settled for the greater good of Homeopathy. Hering benefitted by having its own twenty-bed hospital, while benefitting from Dunham's fine homeopathic library. 1n 1904, further integration took place, with Hering merging with the Hahnemann medical college in Chicago. It was thought that concentrating homeopathy in one distinguished teaching institution in the city would guarantee its viability and hence, ultimate survival. Hering records show JML as professor of physiology as well as graduating as an MD (Hering).[19] In fact Flexner was "brutally frank" and condemnatory about all so-called 'sectarian medical schools' including osteopathic and homeopathic. He criticised their lack of facilities and total inadequacy of their laboratories and dissection rooms. Within a decade of Flexner's report the majority of homeopathic medical schools (including the Hering/Hahnemann in Chicago) had disappeared altogether, only two in New York and Philadelphia survived through to the 1920s.[20]

But let us return to 1900, to the Littlejohn brothers setting up their own osteopathic college. They found a suitable building at 405 West Washington Boulevard, Chicago, and called it the American College of Osteopathic Medicine and Surgery (ACOM & S). JML became its head, President, and professor of Physiology and also, Osteopathy. James, possibly also treasurer[21], made certain that Materia Medica was taught throughout, whilst he was professor of Surgery, Gynaecology and Obstetrics. Finally, David was secretary, as well as Professor of Chemistry, Urinalysis and Public Health.[22] [23] It ran as a two year course, combining osteopathy and surgery. Additionally, its graduates could attend a postgraduate course in major surgery. The college's clinical training was carried out at Cook County hospital, an extremely important well-run facility with a wide spectrum of clinical cases.[24] At some stage within the first years, the college transferred to 495-7 West Monroe Street, Chicago, 3 miles west of its former site. The rival Chicago College of Osteopathy, possibly unable to remain viable with an insufficient number of students, merged with the American College in 1903. By this time the course had been extended to three years, while the postgraduate course on major surgery became a fourth year for those wishing to study. By 1905, 114 students had graduated, plus a further 6 in major surgery.[25]

Meanwhile, JML had further advanced his ideas on his osteopathic fundamental precepts. He affirmed a set of principles very much at the heart of A T Still's early ideas, namely that dysfunction was the source of some illnesses but also at the centre was dysfunction's affect on the individual. This JML considered was explained through physiology, "Hyper physiology", within a person. When the body or mind was unable to adjust to these circumstances then this 'maladjustment' occurred, which had to be rectified to prevent further repercussions on a person's health. The job of an osteopath was to discover these maladjustments, be they structural, work-related, environmental, dietetic or psychological. Furthermore, JML's hypothesis went beyond Still's accepted precepts. JML hypothesised that a person's symptoms were the superficial presentation of a much deeper underlying maladjustment/maladaptive dysfunction. Still's idea, simplified by others, that a spinal bone out of place was the source of much illness made no sense to many outside the profession and raised eyebrows to some within. Traditionalists held on to ideas supported decades later by credible research undertaken by J Stedman Denslow and Irwin Korr in the 1940s and 1950s, concerning substantive evidence of a spinal lesion. Although their work has been the high point of osteopathic enquiry, they arrived at two fundamental questions: what is the spinal lesion's effect on disease and how can its removal by manipulation effect a disease's outcome? They were never able to resolve this conundrum.[26] Moreover, this pursuit of spinal lesions and that of curative manipulative dexterity appeared to critics as pointless snake-oil rationale and remedies.

JML's hypothesis, neodarwinian in concept, suggested individuals within our species who failed to adapt or adjust to life's changes were vulnerable to suffer general health dysfunction at some point in life. It seemed reasonable: a simple explanation of how certain psycho-social factors can influence ill-health. However, this was condemned by a majority of osteopathic colleagues as tantamount to heresy.[27] A T Still in his dotage must have wished inwardly that he had expressed these views, or that others had interpreted his principles in a broader fashion. In a sense, JML in Chicago was freed from the shackles of suppressing his opinions for the sake of not offending the Still family. He turned Still's "structure governs function" around to suggest the opposite: function not only influences structure but the whole organism. He also suggested that the defence mechanisms of the body can be bolstered to aid healing.

These notions appear to come from sources outside osteopathy, and we need look no further than his homeopathic influences.

More importantly, his involvement with both Dunham and Hering Homeopathic schools possibly enabled him to think beyond the confined clinical areas of his osteopathic colleagues. His disadvantage would be that he could not convince his colleagues nor express his views in a clear succinct way for them to understand and support him. To the rescue came his devoted student, E S Comstock, a distinguished colleague from the Littlejohn College alumni, with a clarity and understanding of Littlejohn's lectures on osteopathic principles. Comstock wrote lucidly and debated effectively by presenting these concepts in a more coherent way than the master himself.[28] Another graduate, Dr. Flora Swengel, a graduate of the class of '08, stated "Dr J (JML) was a great teacher, but I never seemed to know how or what to ask him, lest I make a mistake. I think the distance between my brain power and his was just too great."[29] Many future students and graduates at the BSO would have said amen to those words.

Swengel also noted that his brother "Dr J B (James) was a great surgeon and a wonderful teacher. He somehow made us want to ask questions and helped us to understand the answers. He was usually quick to answer, but always seemed relaxed. I cannot remember anyone ever went to sleep in his class; we were too afraid of missing an interesting point. I thought he could do more things at one time than anyone I ever knew."[30] James was well supported by his wife, Edith Mary Williams, an osteopathic physician, who participated on the Littlejohn College of Osteopathy board of management committee, starting in 1904 after David's resignation from the board. She played a crucial role in that capacity for many years. [31] (By contrast Mabel, J Martin's wife, lived a traditional maternal role, bringing up the family and running their modest home in Lake Bluff.[32]) Edith was an osteopathic physician who had additional administrative skills, which she used to great effect at college meetings supporting her husband. Moreover she was aware of James's increasing influence among staff and students.

In 1904 youngest brother David lost interest in osteopathy and the Chicago College by enlisting on a course in law, but kept up his teaching and public health interests.[33] He appears to have had little real interest in osteopathy after leaving Kirksville but probably continued to go along with his two brothers until his resignation from the board of

Directors sometime between 1902-1904.[34] His attitude might well have been influenced by his eldest brother, William, who had undertaken an orthodox medical training, rather dismissing osteopathy altogether. Whether JML and his brother James bought out David's share of the college is not known, but by 1908 their mother Elizabeth had been appointed a director of the college.[35]

Things appeared to be proceeding undramatically until 1909: firstly the college charter from1902 was amended to become the Littlejohn College and Hospital, and secondly its building was redesigned and enlarged to cope with a greater number of students.[36] At the same time the college, possibly under the instigation of James Littlejohn, decide to promote an extended teaching of Materia Medica, (that is the prescribing of drugs), to the curriculum.

This was highlighted by the Illinois State Board of Health issuing three different licences to practice. The most prestigious was for Physicians and Surgeons, the next one for 'drugless practitioners' and the least valuable licence was for midwives. The worthiest licence required that school training should include a state Board of Health-approved medical course embracing a proficient materia medica. The Littlejohn College of Osteopathy (LCC) duly applied for State Board recognition, but failed on inspection as being 'inadequately taught'. Whilst going through their Flexner Inspection, the Littlejohn brothers pursued yet another application for the Littlejohn College of Osteopathy's materia medica and pharmacology course.

It was the publication of Abraham Flexner's 1910 report on the state of North American and Canadian medical schools that would have such a profound effect not only on their own school's relative status but also the direction which those schools would take during the 20th century.

Flexner and his co-workers inspected the Littlejohn College of Osteopathy in December 1909. Clearly they were not impressed. In his report he rather dismisses it as "an undisguised commercial enterprise" and under laboratory facilities continues, "Practically none. At the time of the visit, some rebuilding was in progress, in consequence of which even such laboratories *as are claimed* (my italics) were, except that of elementary chemistry, entirely out of commission and likely to remain so for months: but 'teaching goes on all the same.' "...(the Littlejohn college) has lately in rebuilding wrecked all its laboratories but that of Chemistry without in the least interfering with its usual pedagogic routine".[37] Classrooms were practically bare, except for chairs and a table. Perhaps Flexner was suggesting that these supposed laboratories never actually existed. As for its hospital, he considers, "a pay institution of 20 beds, mostly surgical, can be of little use". [38]

Furthermore in his report on Illinois he states, "The city of Chicago in respect to medical education is the plague spot of the country." He points out the limitations of Cook County Hospital as a training resource for some Chicago medical schools including the Littlejohn. Although he compliments the hospital on its broad spectrum of diseases treated there, he cites a dispute between nurses and rather arrogant medical staff who carelessly ruffle the bedclothes of patients while doing their ward rounds with students. Clearly, the nurses won a notable victory over their medical colleagues, which led to the banning of all medical students from its wards and restricting them to a few exhibition rooms to inspect specific patients. Meanwhile, Flexner cautioned medical staff and medical students to realise that privileges and courtesies go hand in hand and should not be taken for granted. He concluded that such limitations on their clinical training would be to their detriment on graduation. Additionally, none of the outlying hospitals contained the wide spectrum of cases exemplified in Cook County Hospital.[39]

Although eight osteopathic colleges had welcomed their inclusion in the Flexner report on medical schools, many colleagues perceived that it was an anathema, very much against A T Still's traditional anti drug and anti surgical concepts, to be considered comparable. Even in Peoria, Illinois, one DO who had twin MD qualifications was forced to resign his AOA membership for prescribing drugs.

J Martin and James Littlejohn had continuously striven to upgrade their college standards by initiating a third year of study in 1904 and later a further fourth year in1911. Frustratingly they were being squeezed on both sides: by colleagues suspicious that their true intentions were to turn the college into a bona fide MD school and by the Illinois State Medical Association wielding unnecessary influence on the State Board of Health to defer all attempts by them for full licence to practice.[40] The Littlejohn brothers again went for litigation against the State Board but subsequently lost the case. [41] After the court case provisionally materia medica was struck off the list of subjects taught.[42]

Meanwhile J Martin Littlejohn had written to the *Chicago Daily Tribune* denying that Flexner or any of 'his confreres' had inspected the college.

An interesting point of view given that Flexner details an accurate description of the school and its deficient facilities in his report. Furthermore, the osteopathic myth persists today not only in Chicago but also in Flexner's inspection of the ASO, that Kirksville never took place.[43] The historic reaction among osteopaths to Flexner's Report was a yearning to return to a supposed golden traditional era. But in reality it was a period of vigorous competition from a vibrant emerging chiropractic. The osteopathic profession was caught between a hostile medical opposition and an evangelical chiropractic rival.

Further setbacks occurred when the AOA, dominated by 'traditionalists', threatened to renege on LCO accreditation as an affiliated college.[44] Additionally, LCO alumni opposing any extension of the curriculum petitioned Carl McConnell and other Chicago colleagues to support notions of returning to a more traditional based course. Osteopathy worked well and more effectively if the osteopath and his or her patient believed in its therapeutic powers. Within this osteopathic ghetto it provided a degree of awe and respect, but outside this domain, apathy, suspicion and hostility. Indeed, E S Comstock had written an article in the *Journal of the American Osteopathic Association* in defence of J Martin Littlejohn's "universal " principles of adjustment and adaptation which facilitate good health. It was heavily criticised and rebuked by leaders of the profession.[45]

Meanwhile, during the fall of 1912, senior members of the LCO faculty, including Fred Bishoff, Edgar Comstock, Charles Fink and Ernest Proctor, held a number of meetings with James Littlejohn to discuss reorganising the school, with the title of Chicago College of Osteopathy (CCO), under a board of independent trustees.[46] Whereas the AOA had been critical of Flexner's Report, it conceded that colleges could be controlled through an independent board of trustees. These local discussions culminated with a gathering of colleagues at Carl McConnell's office in October. During the meeting, a committee consisting of Bishoff, Comstock, Proctor and Fink, was appointed by those present to initiate a set of proposals to reform the college and its structure.[47] The sequence of events is somewhat obscure. However, we do know that around this time some of the college faculty not only envisaged a root and branch reform but a change of leadership too. It is thought that JML was asked to apply for presidency of the new college in order to engineer his demise as head, a proviso to prevent his automatic reappointment. There were at least two candidates including JML put forward, but the favoured candidate was James, his brother.

This was a bitter pill for JML to swallow, not only was he usurped from his presidency but by his own younger brother to boot. This whole episode has been erased from CCO records, but the repercussions within the Littlejohn family have haunted them for decades. J Martin made haste to leave the USA with his wife and six young children, renounce his American citizenship and never to return to its shores. He never forgave James for what he perceived as fraternal disloyalty, and for supposedly plotting his end as president. Edith's influence to further her husband James was critical during this time. Her experience on the board of management gave her a pivotal, decisive and supportive role during this struggle.

The reality was that J Martin was never quite able to affirm solid support from colleagues in advancing his cause, especially after their wholesale rejection of his hypothesis away from the spinal lesion. Nor did he even quite understand James' superior standing among the faculty and students. Furthermore, both Littlejohns failed in their final application attempt for full medical and surgical licence for the college, due to the resoluteness of the Illinois state medical board's opposition. The time for fraternal cooperation in collegiate matters came to an end. James and Martin never communicated again. The sale of the Littlejohn College and Hospital to a new board was controlled by James and Edith Littlejohn as the newly inducted LCO president and secretary respectively. On the 4th February 1913, 65 osteopathic colleagues met in Mrs Ellis' Tea Room to form a new Illinois osteopathic association, to elect seven independent trustees and to rename the college under a revised charter, the "Chicago College of Osteopathy". The CCO emphasised a more traditional osteopathic ethos by dropping materia medica and pharmacology from the curriculum and relinquishing all efforts for Illinois State accreditation as a medical school. It was only in 1955 that the CCO gained full medical licence.[48]

JML was dismissed thus for a second time in his brief osteopathic teaching career, once as dean of Kirksville and now as President of the Chicago college. Perhaps his situation was exacerbated by his inability to deliver his ideas succinctly and clearly enough to students and colleagues, unlike his brother James.[49] In the end, his failure to persuade them of his advanced thesis on adaptation/adjustment resulted in his dismissal.

Perhaps his notions could have determined a third way for osteopathic direction? But, sadly, they were irretrievably set aside, never to become central to his teaching at his British School of Osteopathy either.

This clarion call never came for adopting his neodarwinian idea, that when an individual is unable to adapt to events then general health dysfunction can occur. It is a measure of failure on his part not to persist with it and on his profession for not recognizing its value. In a couple of decades, sulphonamides (precursors of antibiotics) would emerge in the eternal struggle against acute and sub acute episodes of infectious diseases. Fifty years ago notions of adaptation/adjustment to life changes would have been perceived by parents, relations, friends, colleagues and a hostile corpus of orthodox medical practitioners as reckless. Nevertheless, their importance as a major factor of chronic illness became more apparent, and acute conditions treated with antibiotics were less effective. The unremitting mutation of hostile bugs and the waning effectiveness of antibiotics in countering infection make the human race vulnerable to pandemics in the twenty first century and beyond.

---

1   Caskey M J *A History of Amity College* Chicago College of Osteopathic Medicine (CCOM) archives p.10. *David Littlejohn* CCM archives p.2. There is some doubt about David's medical qualifications: his time at central medical school, St Joseph's Michigan 1897-1898 appears too short. We can assume that his brother J Martin was not the only brother to embellish his qualifications. David appears to promote his B Ph (Amity College) to PhD but there is doubt about his medical qualifications too.
2   NOA. Scanned material. J M Littlejohn further documents. *Littlejohn depositions 100.*pp. 3, 33, 38..
3   Collins M. *Osteopathy in Britain*. Booksurge. 2005. p.42.
4   Flexner A. *Medical Education in the United States and Canada: A Report to the Carnegie Foundation for the Advancement of Teaching*. The Carnegie Foundation. 1910. pp. 253-4.
5   Trowbridge C. *Andrew Taylor Still 1828-1917*. Truman State University Press. 1991. p. 174. Interestingly, there is no knowledge of its existence in Flexner's Report of 1910.
6   *Biography of David Littlejohn* Archives CCOM p.1
7   NOA. DVD and CD Archive *Anne and Sara Kennard Interview*. 2010. DVD
8   Trowbridge C. p.214
9   Ibid p. 214
10 Gevitz N. *The DO's: Osteopathic Medicine in America*. The John Hopkins University Press. 1982 . p.79.
11 Campbell E A letter to Ken Morgan, CCOM, CCOM archives 7 December 1993 p.1
12 Kennard, Anne and Sara "conversation on JML and Mabel 29th September 2014
13 NOA. Scanned material. Further J M Littlejohn further documents. Waring G.P. *History of Dunham Medical School*. Edited by W H King *The History of Homeopathy and Its Institutions in America* . The Lewis Publishing Co. New York and Chicago. 1905 Volume III. Chapter 3. pp .3-4

14 House of Lords, Select Committee of the. *Registration and Regulation of Osteopaths Bill.* London: H.M. Stationery Office, 1935.p.230 nos. 3505-3517.
15 NOA. Scanned material. Further J M Littlejohn further documents. Waring G.P. p.6
16 Still C E to Dr Earnest Roberts of Harrogate, Yorkshire, England 23 March 1900. NOA. J Martin Littlejohn archive file box 2 Letter from
17 Waring G.P. pp.1-2
18 ibid p.3 and p.6
19 Allen H.C. & King J.B.S. *Hering Medical College and Hospital;* Edited by W H King *The History of Homeopathy and Its Institutions in America.* The Lewis Publishing Co. New York and Chicago. 1905 Volume II Chapter XV pp.431-434.
20 Kaufman M. *Homeopathy in America* edited by N. Gevitz *Other Healers: Unorthodox Medicine in America* John Hopkins University Press Baltimore & London 1988. pp.111-112.
21 ACOM & S Board of Directors 1904, CCOM archives shows James was both ACOM& S treasurer& secretary, following David's resignation as secretary.
22 *Littlejohn Dispositions 1900* pp.2;29;35.
23 *Chicago City Directories* notes Chicago College of Osteopathic Medicine Archives
24 Flexner A. p.218.
25 Booth E.R. *History of Osteopathy* Caxton Press: Cincinnati. 1905 pp.93-94.
26 Gevitz N. *The DOs* pp.90-92
27 Comstock E S *"The Littlejohn College Idea"* Journal of The American Osteopathic Association (JAOA) 11 (1911): 656-76; *"A Letter from Dr. Littlejohn"* JAOA 11 (1911): 727-729.
28 Hall T E *The Contribution of John Martin Littlejohn to Osteopathy* The Osteopathic Publishing Company Ltd 1952 pp.25-27.
29 Berchtold T., *To Teach, To Heal, To Serve! A History of the Chicago College of Osteopathic Medicine 1900-1975* Chicago: Chicago College of Osteopathic Medicine, 1975 p.16.
30 ibid pp.16-17
31 Board of Directors, ACOM & S 1904-5 Booklet, CCOM archives
32 Forlow, D. Local historian Lake Bluff. Correspondence by email 19-07-2012 (Copies held in NOA. J Martin Littlejohn archive)
33 *Biography of David Littlejohn* CCOM Archives p.1
34 *American College of Osteopathic Medicine & Surgery Prospectus* 1904 p.8
35 *American College of Osteopathic Medicine & Surgery Prospectus* 1908
36 Comstock E S Chicago College of Osteopathy: Its History *Reflex* 1923 p.91
37 ibid. p.214
38 Flexner A. pp.214-5
39 ibid pp.218-9
40 Gevitz N Osteopathic Medicine in Chicago: 1900-1985; *Proc. Inst. Med. Chicago.* Vol. 38. 1985 p.153.
41 Gevitz N. *The DOs* pp.69-70
42 Gevitz N. *Other Healers* p.137 He also suggests that the college changed hands but this appears to be 3 years ahead of time.
43 Littlejohn J.M. *Chicago Daily Tribune* 8th June 1910 p.6.
44 Gevitz N. Osteopathic Medicine in Chicago: 1900-1985 p.154
45 Hall T.E. pp.34-36
46 Littlejohn J B *Chicago College of Osteopathy* Magazine 1939 Edition p.16
47 Comstock E S Chicago College of Osteopathy: Its History *Reflex* 1923 p.91
48 Gevitz N. Osteopathic Medicine in Chicago: 1900-1985 p.154
49 Berchtold T. pp.16-17

Chapter 4
Those degrees, doctorates and visits: return to Britain

In his memorable Littlejohn lecture in 1952, T Edward Hall wonders about J Martin's degrees ascribed in the front of his thesis published in 1895. He deduces that some are just American variations of his Glasgow degrees but that he cannot understand FNU or FCC. We know now that they refer to his time at Columbia College (FCC – Fellow of Columbia College, New York) and the National Night University (FNNU, not FNU, Fellow of National Night University, Chicago).[1] This is a period when JML departed from his previous standards of academic honours to accumulate qualifications of dubious origin and consideration. Some say that he perceived them as rather irrelevant chattels, but this goes against the evidence. He acquired them as an eager scout accumulates badges to display proudly on his uniform. This interest in accumulating dubious doctorates found some resonance in his visit to England at the end of the Kirksville academic year of 1898.

In July of that year, he gave a paper on "Osteopathy in line of apostolic succession with Medicine" to a quasi-respectable Society of Science, Letters and Arts at the Addison Hall, London. This was a nomadic, rather tenuous organisation, meeting at various venues, in existence for a number years, but never having a base. Be that as it may, JML's presentation was considered a success, being awarded a Gold medal for his lecture.[2] At some stage, he had either become a member or was invited to join the society, and used its letters FSScLA, preferring to shorten them to Fellow of the Society of Science, FSSc. He used them, as did his brothers David and James also utilise these letters,[3] as part of a ribbon of degrees and qualifications for all three to impress the Still family and fellow faculty members during their time at Kirksville and, later, Chicago. This was tantamount, as Sir William Jowitt retorted during the select committee report on *The Registration and Regulation of Osteopaths Bill* (1935), to paying one's membership fees to the Royal Geographical Society or London Zoo and using FRGS or FZS respectively after your name as a professional qualification and academic honour. In any case, there was no need to have done it, given his possession of worthy Glaswegian academic awards.[4] Nevertheless, he made another trip to London the following year to give a second lecture to the Society of Science, Letters and Arts. This time the subject was entitled "Osteopathy as a Science". During this visit he enrolled as a member of the Royal Society of Literature too, and appended its letters, FRSL (Fellow of the Royal Society of Literature) to his list of other awards.[5]

On returning to America it was erroneously reported that he had addressed the Royal Society of Science (having attached a 'Royal' prefix to its title) rather than simply the Society of Science, Letters and Arts at Crystal Palace, London on 19th July 1899. Although the Crystal Palace building was world famous for its exhibition in 1851 at Westminster, central London, it had been transferred three years later to Norwood within its own park, surrounded by Victorian residential developments.[6] It is highly unlikely that JML's lecture took place in the building but in a library in Upper Norwood. Inadvertently, news of his lecture was misconstrued that he had addressed the Royal Society in the prestigious Crystal Palace, the report about it was published as such in the *Journal of Osteopathy*. When Charlie Still investigated this matter further, the event could not be corroborated, nor could his participation as a speaker. By this time, a vendetta between the Still and Littlejohn families was taking place. This matter appeared to consolidate Charlie Still's opinion, "I am thoroughly disgusted with the whole affair, and am almost ready to believe anything (about JML)".[7] However, his lecture to the Society of Science, Letters and Arts did definitely take place during July and his membership of the Royal Society of Literature can be substantiated. It is quite possible that people misconstrued both societies, and there is no proof that JML did not try to explain these events correctly. However, he did appear to exploit the title by using FRSL as an academic award, even dropping the L later to utilise it as FRS, Fellow of the Royal Society, an august society of eminent scientists stretching back to its foundation by King Charles II in the 17th century.[8] Furthermore, JML stated that he was awarded a medal in Physiology by the Royal Society of Science, conveniently dropping 'Letters & Arts' from the title, which rather supports Charlie Still's opinion that JML had lied about his academic engagements.[9] In 1900, JML had left Kirksville under a cloud with his two brothers to settle in Chicago. From there he set off to sail to England for one very important reason.

Chapter 4

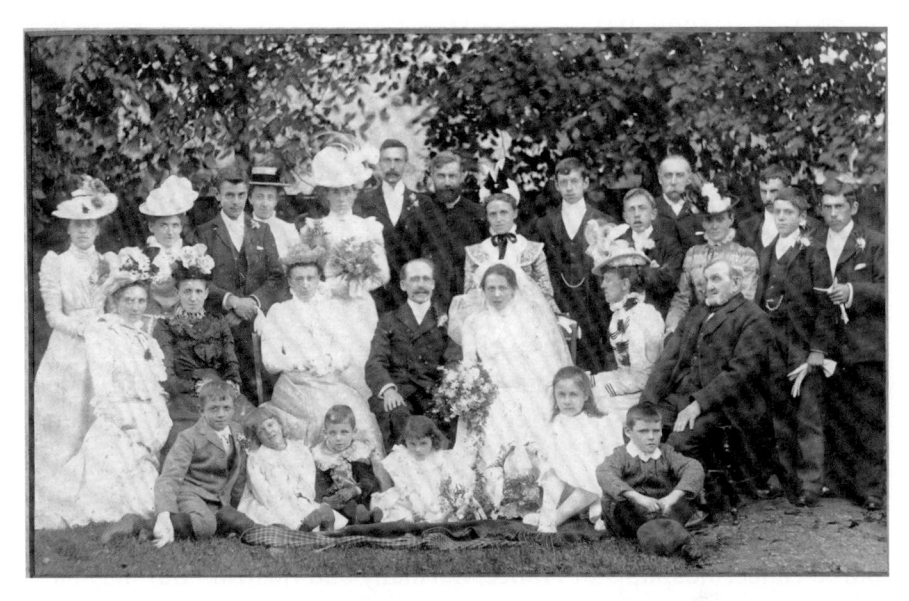

The wedding of JML and Mabel

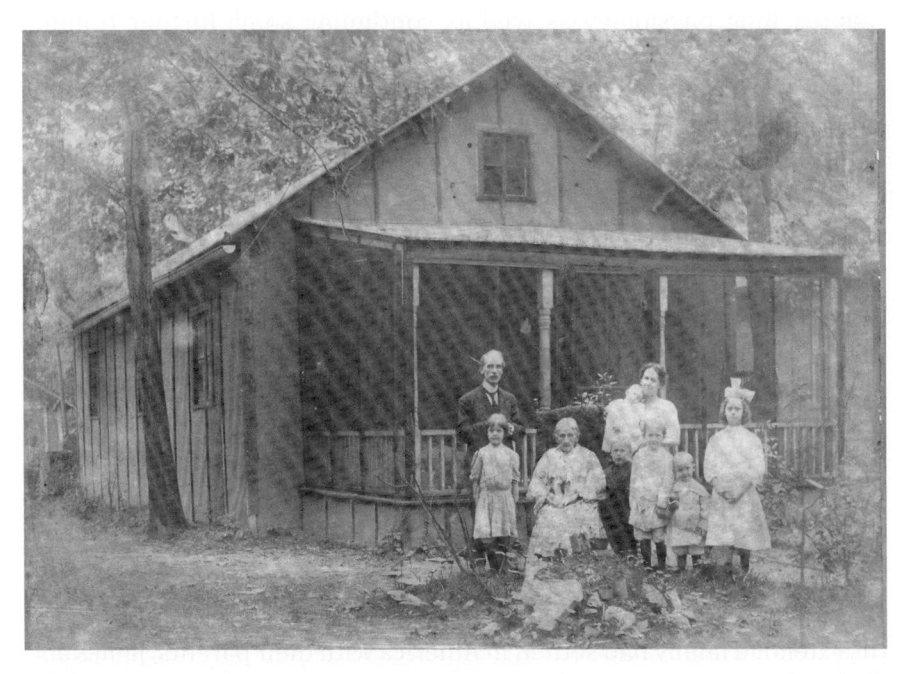

JML, Mabel, mother Elizabeth and the six children at home in Lake Bluff

55

On 7th August 1900, JML married Mabel Alice Thompson at a wedding in Ipswich, Suffolk, England. Whilst there he found time to give a further lecture to the Society of Science, Letters and Arts, "Osteopathy, a new view of the Science of Therapeutics". (He also states in the 1923 edition of *The Reflex,* journal of the Chicago College of Osteopathy, that copies of all three lectures to this society were presented to members of the British Medical Association at its annual General Meeting in 1900.[10] [11]) With his new wife he returned to the USA to settle down to marital life in the prestigious Illinois town of Lake Bluff, 35 miles north of Chicago. Although their home was a fairly modest abode, the neighbourhood contained some large mansions.[12] During their time at Lake Bluff, Mabel gave birth to three boys, all three being associated with his British School of Osteopathy in later life, and three girls.[13]

He made a further visit to Europe and stopped off in Britain in 1903, under the auspices of researching the effects of cancer treatment. He toured cancer hospitals in France, Germany and Austria[14] but may have been, more specifically, visiting homeopathic institutions specialising in cancer treatments. (Appropriately, he had gained his MD degree at Dunham Homeopathic Medical School, Chicago, the previous year, and was teaching physiology as well as continuing some further training at Hering Homeopathic Medical School.) During his time in Britain, he met with Franz Horn (London) and Willard Walker (Scotland), the first osteopaths to practise in the UK, in order to discuss the founding of a British osteopathic school. Subsequently a year later both Jay Dunham and Harvey Foote, practising in Ireland, volunteered to help them establish a college.[15] However,this project was put aside by Littlejohn in order to focus on more immediate considerations back in Chicago.

Although his reputation was in the ascendency outside the influence of the Still family, by 1908 the A T Still Research Institute had appointed him along with C A Whiting as one of three research team leaders - their responsibility being to determine osteopathic effects on neoplasms (cancers).[16] This may have been the high water mark of his achievements in his osteopathic career during his time in America. Four years later, his reputation was in tatters. Shunned by the profession's leaders, his colleagues in Chicago and by his brother James, J Martin Littlejohn assessed his situation.

His extended family had settled in America with their parents, James and Elizabeth, who had died in 1900 and 1911 respectively. They are both buried in Kirksville, Missouri. There is ample evidence that Elizabeth, after their father's death, had lived with various family members around Chicago until her own death.[17] J Martin's eldest brother William had retrained as an orthodox medical physician but never showed any interest in osteopathy. David, who initially did maintain some loyalty towards it, lost his enthusiasm and specialised in public health from 1906 onwards. Brother James had shown that his commitment to osteopathy was sustained, provided that surgery was included in its training and practice. Moreover his interest was consolidated by his wife Edith, a graduate of Kirksville, who supported her husband in all things. With the death of both parents, JML's subsequent falling out with his colleagues and with James, he decided to cut his losses. Financially comfortable from his endeavours, he returned to the UK with his wife Mabel and six young children. However, it is postulated that he never settled a substantial debt to the local store in Lake Bluff before embarking on the SS Corinthian, 29th June 1913.[18]

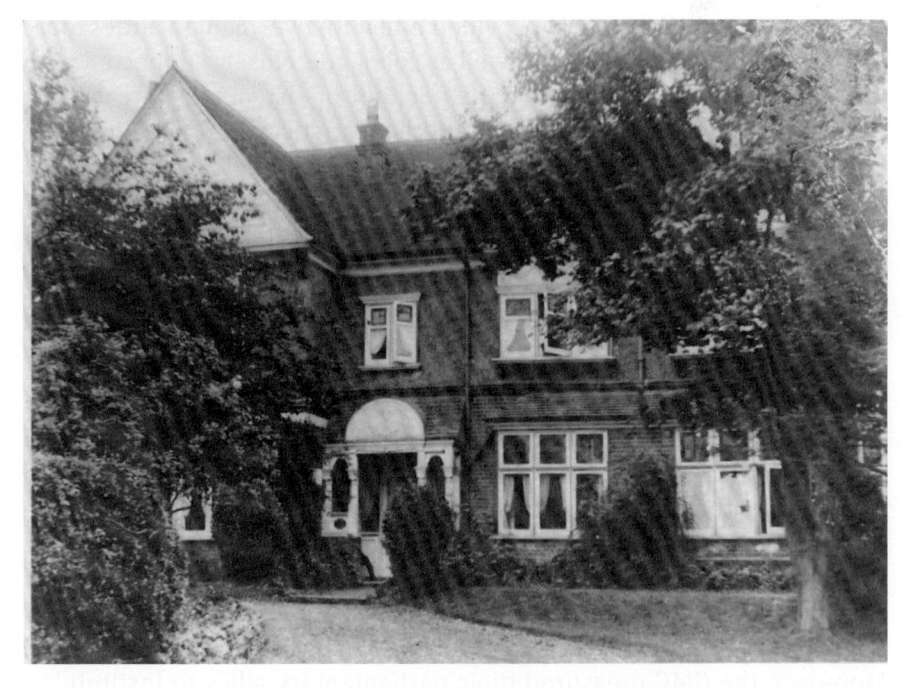

Badger Hall: beloved by JML and family!

The urgency of such a move led to J Martin Littlejohn purchasing (possibly outright and without viewing) Badger Hall, a roomy late Victorian house, with farmworkers' cottages plus outhouses, located in the village of Thundersley, North Benfleet, Essex. It was very rudimentary: without mains drainage, electricity, gas or water. It was typical of most country dwellings - dependent upon oil lamps and candles for lighting, an outside privy or earth closet and water from a well.[19] It had some advantages (much of the surrounding area is on high ground, Canvey island being just 2 miles away was very vulnerable to flooding), especially being located only a half mile from the railway station, with a regular service from South Benfleet to Fenchurch Street, London, a journey of less than an hour. This was ideal for his practice in Piccadilly, a twenty minute bus trip from Fenchurch Street. He shared consulting rooms with two osteopathic sisters, Clara Hough and Mrs J E Hough Collins, together with his friend J Stewart Moore. A few years later it appears that the tenancy lease was at an end and all were forced to find new premises. Subsequently, J Martin Littlejohn and J Stewart Moore transferred to 48 Dover Street, which possibly provided him with overnight facilities too.[20] Moore became a solid friend as well as colleague, closely connected with the formation of Littlejohn's British School of Osteopathy. Meanwhile Littlejohn appears to have opened another practice at 15 The Ridgeway Enfield, which he accessed by rail from Liverpool Street station, and also ran a practice for Southend-on-Sea patients from his home at Badger Hall. These two satellite ventures provided 50 treatments per week at a reduced rate to all.[21]

Before we go any further, we must go back five years to 1908, when osteopaths began to establish practices, especially in central London.

In that year, the medical establishment put their critical spotlight on Herbert Barker, the bonesetters' de facto star, celebrity practitioner and self-publicist. An upsurge in the popularity of British bonesetters had occurred at the same time that this worthy practitioner had become publicly prominent. Sir Herbert Barker's growing eminence continued thanks to some astute publicity.[22] His celebrity status spotlighted him spectacularly to the attention of his orthodox foes. The General Medical Council (GMC) initiated a campaign to impugn Barker and his colleagues. Moreover, the GMC pressured their parliamentary allies to institute an official survey to review "the evil effects produced by the unrestricted practice of medicine and surgery by unqualified persons."[23] Furthermore, a resentful client was exhorted to take Barker to court. In his verdict statement the judge found him guilty of the charges made and only awarded a trivial sum to the plaintiff but with all costs of the case against Barker. This was a considerable amount that could have bankrupted him, and furthermore, his reputation was temporarily damaged too, much to the delight of his medical antagonists. Two years later the parliamentary report on unqualified practitioners was published in 1910.

it provided conclusive proof of what the GMC feared: the report showed that bonesetting had flourished with increasing numbers of practitioners and with its public reputation enhanced. By 1911, the GMC responded by discouraging any medical cooperation with bonesetters by expelling Barker's anaesthetist, Dr W F Axham, from its register, for "infamous conduct".[24] This fait accompli appeared to victimise a distinguished elderly medical practitioner and its action created a public backlash, with the GMC being branded as heavyhanded bully boys. Outrage was voiced in the press, including in *The Times,* (which invariably supported orthodox medicine), its editorial described Barker as "having effected perfect cures where regular surgeons had failed."[25] This incident produced a twofold reaction from the GMC: no other medical practitioner was ever struck off or penalised for professionally assisting a bonesetter or osteopath. Needless to say some reprimands and threats were indirectly made to doctors during subsequent decades, but no punishment meted out; and Barker's damaged reputation, practice and finances were triumphantly fully restored.

Just as Barker had won a significant victory over his medical opponents, the popularity of bonesetters had reached its zenith before waning rapidly as naturopathy, osteopathy and chiropractic infiltrated their areas of skill and their potential market. Bonesetting's weakness in the UK and vulnerability are explained by its variable training within apprenticeships and negligible trade associations. The beneficiaries were chiropractors and osteopaths, their biophysical concepts and terminology were not dissimilar. Although British chiropractic and osteopathic colleges were rudimentary, fragile institutions, they laid down a way forward in training that bonesetting ignored at its cost. Moreover, during this time, practitioners of osteopathy, chiropractic and naturopathy began to organise themselves into cohesive elementary groups.

Following Barker's confrontation with the British medical establishment, on 1st July 1911 the British Osteopathic Society (BOS)[26] was formed to protect and foster activities of those osteopaths trained under American college accreditation with the American Osteopathic Association (AOA). The BOS had been co-founded by Dr Hudson who was "conscious of the strenuous medical opposition" and believed "it was time for (American trained) osteopaths to form a distinctive organisation."[27] This particular group was moving professionally and socially, like Barker, among the country's elite, members of the establishment, and high society in central London. J Martin Littlejohn became a member two years later on settling in England and took a relatively active part from the start.[28]

Interests of bonesetters and osteopaths coincided when attending wounded combatants of World War One. Both made a number of entreaties to the War Office for official recognition to treat casualties, but these were refused. The War Office responded by rather pompously quoting King's regulations, which prevented the official employ of any unregistered medical practitioner. Consequently both groups bypassed this red tape and treated various military personnel privately, many without ever charging a fee. In 1917 Noel Buxton MP cited in the House of Commons the excellent war work attributed to Bonesetters and Osteopaths[29] and also made a proposal through political channels to overturn "these anomalous conditions".[30] Although this attempt to change the King's regulations was futile, belated official appreciation was bestowed on Barker (in 1922 he was knighted for his manipulative services to the royal family and the establishment),[31] and, following successful political lobbying, osteopaths were also given public approval.[32] Meanwhile some sympathetic orthodox doctors were prepared to ignore medical authorities' threats and work alongside the bonesetters and osteopaths.

Several years later the GMC returned to this familiar theme, namely that any anaesthetists cooperating with "unregistered persons" were cautioned against ignoring this directive, with the threat of their "name erased from the Medical Register".[33] Although this had some deterrent effect from assisting bonesetters and osteopaths, others remained adamant in disregarding such a ruling and continued to associate themselves. In 1924, The American osteopath Wilfrid Streeter founded the Osteopathic Defence League (ODL), a group of sympathetic influential lay-persons, to counter these GMC intimidations and appeal for statutory regulation. Meanwhile, Sir Herbert Barker became a resolute ally, and publicly petitioned its cause. Streeter was heartened by Barker's resoluteness, and in a quid pro quo gesture, secured an honorary doctorate (DO) for him from his alma mater the American School of Osteopathy.[34] Furthermore, Streeter's friend, Arthur Greenwood MP, decided to question the GMC's prejudicial attitude in the House of Commons.

Meanwhile, Littlejohn's plan to organise a British osteopathic training establishment was carried out by himself and Franz Horn in 1917 when the British School of Osteopathy (BSO) was incorporated. (Littlejohn writes later about the school having some sort of existence two years before this event, but this was largely focused on his establishment of clinics during the Great War for the benefit of wounded service personnel.) The origins of the BSO are quite obscure, its gestation period being quite prolonged. We know that he appointed his friend and colleague J Stewart Moore as clinic superintendent in 1922 and together with another colleague William Cooper became a member of the BSO Council of Education and BSO director (1924-6). However, these actions do not inform us when the first students enrolled for osteopathic training. It is more likely that the original class was peripatetically located in a number of places, including Littlejohn's and Stewart Moore's own consulting rooms in Dover Street, before settling in Franz Horn's House, free of charge, in Vincent Square, London in 1925.[35]

At this time Horn, Moore and Cooper probably held Littlejohn in high esteem, for he had been appointed BOA President (1925-6). Its council was drawing up plans to publicly announce a BOA manifesto setting out its main strategy to head British manipulative practice, irrespective of any medical professional involvement or any other non-medical interested grouping. This was a blunt naïve idea, completely oblivious to the gathering opposition engendered by such ill-thought and outlandish proposals. Be that as it may, the manifesto was launched at the Palace of Westminster on 31st March 1925 by the BOA's undoubted star, Kelman MacDonald, osteopath and consultant physician, to a parliamentary audience consisting of members of both Houses.

Macdonald outlined a one-sided approved History of Osteopathy: its central principles, its growth in America and its future direction. He cautioned against UK osteopathic courses, other than those of the British School of Osteopathy (BSO), which he stated would provide the necessary training for undergraduate students and postgraduate doctors. He proposed that the BOA would act as an alumnal association for both groups. It was a rather longwinded speech, giving a somewhat rose-tinted, spirited view of osteopathy. But he stressed realistically that osteopathy was a healing *art*, its scientific appreciation would be realised from critical scrutiny and assessment at a later date.[36]

True to its commitment in the manifesto the British Osteopathic Association (BOA), loosely associated to its parent body, the American Osteopathic Association (AOA), accepted the first cohort of BSO graduates, Elsie Wareing and Gerald Lowry, as full association members. Meanwhile, the BSO was accredited, and further support was shown by 11 BOA members joining the BSO faculty as part-time staff.[37] The role of the school was to train undergraduates over a four-year period and for medical graduates to undergo a specialised, a one-year course.

However, in early 1926 this convivial state of affairs took on a significantly different tone. J Martin Littlejohn, President of the BOA but also dean of the BSO, met a BOA delegation which was concluding a satisfactory inspection of the school. Their message offered not only a favourable opinion to its inspection but also an ominous directive. School accreditation and alumnal acceptance into BOA membership could only be fulfilled with school control transferred to an independent board of trustees, similar to other AOA accredited schools, according to Flexner's basic requirements for evolving medical education. J Martin's resolute steadfastness was unequivocal, he refused point blank to entertain such an order. His downright obstinacy to countenance such an edict was seen by BOA officials as arrogant and foolhardy.[38] Furthermore, this event resonated from similar episodes during his final years in Chicago: specifically, his demise among colleagues who rejected outright his revision of Still's osteopathic principles, and his rivalry with brother James over the appointment of Carl McConnell to the headship of the newly founded Chicago College of Osteopathy. Additionally, he probably regarded the BSO as a useful form of income: fees from students and those attending BSO student clinics were similar to sums attained during his time at Chicago.

Be that as it may, he was left in no doubt by the BOA delegation that failure to transfer control would lead to BOA sanctions outlined in the meeting, leaving the school and alumni isolated from its AOA parent organisation. A final attempt was made by the BOA in September 1926 to persuade JML to accede to a BOA independent board of trustees, with no result.[39] His continued intransigence left the BOA Council with no room for manoeuvre. It had little choice but to impose penalties on the BSO and its graduates:- the school could not be accredited by the BOA nor the AOA; BOA membership would be refused to all future BSO alumni; and thereby deprive them of association with their American colleagues. The BSO prospectus the following year shows all eleven BOA lecturers missing.[40] No further BSO graduates ever joined the BOA, and AOA accreditation was refused. Consequently in response Littlejohn resigned as BOA President and he forfeited his membership. One member though, Ray Harvey Foote, gave Littlejohn solid support throughout the increasing vitriol between the two institutions, his loyalty and commitment remained constant.

This conflict caused irreparable damage to British osteopathy, separating it away from its American counterpart, and leaving it to develop independently. The BOA sought to distance itself from Littlejohn and the BSO by ignoring its presence. As Shilton Webster-Jones, the former BSO principal, stated, "the BOA rather preferred osteopathic evolution in Britain to progress through official channels but Littlejohn pronounced that it would be by acceptance from public consensus". Although George Bernard Shaw the playwright and Elmer Pheils a Birmingham osteopath were neighbours, Shaw had shown little interest in osteopathy. In 1927, Pheils persuaded Shaw to open the BOA Clinic in central London.[41] `He only did so to irritate the medical profession further'. Meanwhile, Littlejohn had other distractions coming from the North of England.

William Looker, founder and principal of the School of Bloodless Surgery, Manchester, later called the Looker College of Osteopathy and Chiropractic, had died unexpectedly. A number of his students went to the Incorporated Association of Osteopaths (IAO) for assistance to finish their courses, abruptly terminated on his death. The IAO had been formed by a number of Looker graduates only a year before, largely brought about as a response to oppose the BOA manifesto. However, the IAO was a club for those osteopaths looking for convivial meetings, professional chitchat interspersed with the odd talk and discussion. It was not a robust institution willing to metamorphose into a college. Besides, the association could ill afford to shoulder Looker's liabilities which would compromise individual IAO members, consequently none showed zest or inclination to do so. However, they did recommend that the students contact J Martin Littlejohn at the BSO for assistance.

The full effects of the BOA's withdrawal from any support of the BSO and its alumni was starting to dawn on Littlejohn. Deserted by his

BOA colleagues, resigning from the BSO faculty, he was responsible for financing the BSO and taking on the burden of most lectures until sufficient numbers of his own BSO graduates had joined the school faculty. The Looker student appeal for help came out of the blue and appeared as a bonus in a stark year. He welcomed the twelve students, naming them the apostles, and enabling them to complete their training under the auspices of the BSO in a year (He eased their assimilation by awarding them each three years credit for study at the Looker school, even though some critics believed the Looker course to be less than six months duration). Positive news of his favourable treatment towards the apostles reached IAO members and other former Looker graduates. Gradually, further contact was made with Littlejohn, and a number of IAO officials travelled south to meet up with him to discuss matters of mutual benefit, and common to both was an animosity towards the BOA.

When the twelve apostles graduated from the BSO and set up practice in Lancashire and elsewhere in the north of England, they had a choice to join the London-based BSO alumnal the Association of British Osteopaths, or the northern-based IAO. Some Looker graduates and IAO members were anxious to augment their own training under the auspices of the BSO. IAO members agreed to submit to a year's study (July 1927-8) supervised by a member of the BSO faculty through viva voce and 'clinical demonstrations', although they refused to countenance written exams because it was thought "they would, by so doing, forfeit their position as a corporation".[42] Accordingly, Littlejohn awarded them BSO diplomas at the end of their studies. Whether the non-requirement of obligatory written exams was a concession too far is a moot point. In the unyielding light of severe cross-examination by British Medical Association counsel at the House of Lords select committee Osteopaths Bill in 1935, this episode of compromising to lower standards of examination and acceptance of three years credit to Looker students would return to haunt Littlejohn. His answers in reply would reflect disastrously on his tenure at the BSO.[43]

By 1929 the BSO graduate association was absorbed into the IAO. Littlejohn's laissez-faire attitude towards granting BSO diplomas continued with another cohort of students and graduates of the Western School of Osteopathy and British Chiropractic College. Similarly to the IAO situation, they attended the BSO after the simultaneous closure of both establishments. Subsequently these students and graduates were able to join its new professional association, the IAO. Indeed this led to one Western School graduate having a crisis of conscience over his BSO diploma, to be told by Littlejohn not to be troubled but to keep things under wraps.[44]

JML's ability to assist and absorb diverse groups from the north and west of England gave his association more balance, whereas the BOA members were mainly located in central London and the home counties. The BOA, with never more than 80 traditionally trained US members, proceeded to run its own clinic.[45] Though numerically small, their influence on their upper class clientele, plus their close AOA connection, gave them immeasurable power within UK osteopathic institutions. They were top of the osteopathic pecking order. In addition, the BOA members were determined to utilise connections in high places to negotiate certain privileges exclusively for themselves.

Throughout those early years, Littlejohn drove himself relentlessly with a daily programme more suited to a much younger person. Mornings would be spent practising in his Dover Street premises, followed by a walk at lunchtime across Green Park to the BSO at Buckingham Gate. Afternoons were taken up with a heavy load of lectures, to be followed in the early evening with BSO correspondence, before setting off home to Thundersley.

Lack of investment and outside funding meant that the BSO was poorly equipped and stark in appearance. However, this was offset by Littlejohn's driving force and sheer doggedness to promote his vision to students. Moreover, he engendered devotion and a degree of awe among his students, though they may not have quite understood his lectures! He often appeared vague, absent minded and inattentive, and his physical presence could be misconstrued too. His modest frame would be attired in a slightly crumpled suit, "not a credit to his tailor" as one student put it. On occasions during lectures, he nodded off under the strain of all his duties. However, his kindly personality, with its lack of wrath and histrionics, far outweighed most disadvantages. Indeed, he would allow students in financial difficulty to defer payment of their BSO tuition fees. Consequently, he was always out of pocket, some students never paid their dues even after graduation. From within the BSO walls, Littlejohn conveyed studious insights and deep knowledge of his academic subjects, reflected by further warmth and esteem from its student body. From their ranks he selected the most able to join the faculty and clinic in order to lessen his burdensome load and to pass on his essential work to future generations of students.[46] These included the BSO vice-Dean T. Edward Hall, Shilton Webster-Jones, Clem Middleton, Muriel Dunning and, later, Alan Stoddard.

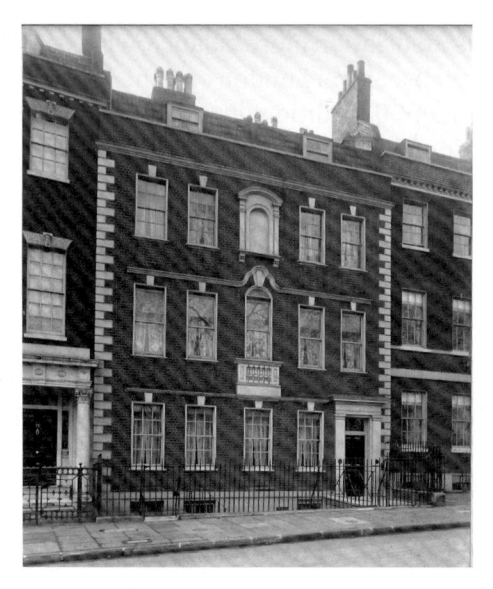

The BSO, 16 Buckingham Gate, London SW1

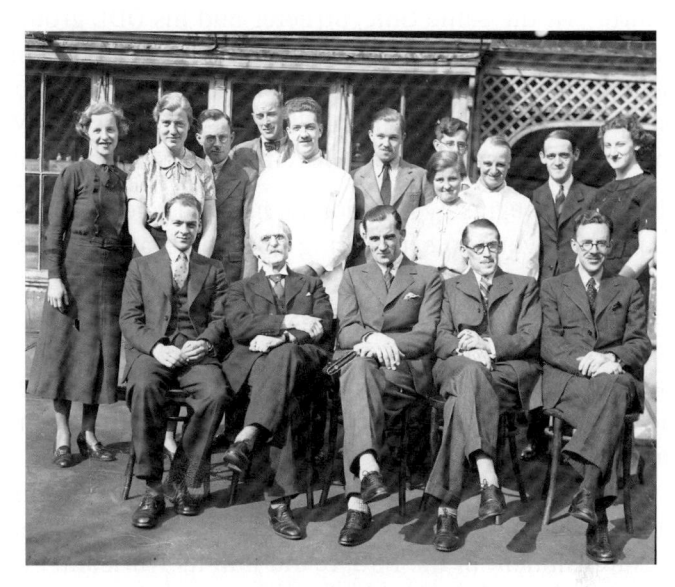

JML and BSO faculty

Sometime during the early 1930s J Martin Littlejohn noted, possibly for future reference, his innermost thoughts on various groups of osteopaths and their relationships with one another. These writings provide clues to the fractious nature of osteopathic institutions with one another. Although they are only his reflections, nevertheless one does gain a fairly accurate impression of the animosity and disdain pervading through rival osteopathic groups. His writings complain how both the BSO and IAO "are consistently ignored by both the BOA and ODL (Osteopathic Defence League)".[47]

He describes how the ODL was founded by Wilfrid Streeter, a US trained American osteopath, as a counterweight, to provide some form of public protection against medical opinion opposed to osteopathy. ODL membership exclusively contained influential lay-people committed to the state regulation of osteopaths. Moreover, Streeter had sought the support and friendship of Sir Herbert Barker, the well-known bonesetter. Streeter flattered Barker by bestowing an honorary doctorate from his alma mater, Kirksville College of Osteopathic Medicine, as a reward for his campaign support. However much he welcomed Barker's interventions to the cause, Streeter rather brushed aside bonesetting as unfinished and unscientific manipulation, whilst osteopathy was the gold standard.[48] At the same time, Streeter and his ODL group publicly disassociated themselves from the BSO, IAO and BOA. Littlejohn wrote –"It was their intention to fight and stand alone" adding "yet expects all three to support (the ODL) whenever it requests to do so".[49] JML's woes did not end with Streeter's ODL, the BOA incurred much disapproval too.

In his writings JML begins by mentioning his own role in 1925-6 as BOA president and his pivotal role in leading a BOA delegation to the Ministry of Health, then headed by the future Prime Minister, Neville Chamberlain MP. Its purpose was to gain the minister's approval for an exclusive Royal Charter for the BOA. It is probable that the party was met by a civil servant who accepted a letter of proposal on behalf of the Minister and in due course, Chamberlain replied to the plea. Littlejohn relates its salient points, "... establish yourselves in the only possible way, get going in School and when 100 students have graduated, apply again and we will consider this application. Having expressly stated that their objects were the establishment of the BSO, to aid it in its work and enable it to become better equipped and to issue diplomas the Minister of Health was extremely far sighted and fair".[50] However, Littlejohn's grievances towards the BOA become apparent.

He berates them for opposing the BSO, cutting off all contact and never setting foot in the BSO. "From that time I have carried the BSO on my shoulders until such time when I have trained my own students to become teachers".[51] He continues in this vein, how BOA members of the faculty resigned, although not mentioning his responsibility for this thanks to his refusal to transfer BSO ownership to an independent board of BOA trustees which gave them no alternative but to leave. He remonstrates in no uncertain manner his alternative view, "no fabulous salaries can be offered" and " because teaching is an art possessed by few". From this position he extols the virtues of the BSO: "how 94 students have graduated since its inception; it has the largest osteopathic clinic treating 20,000 cases; has established affiliated clinics all over the country; has its own school colours and crest; a Students' Union; and Library."[52]

The separation between the BOA and the BSO/IAO practitioners became unbridgeable even when both sides were encouraged to cooperate. JML's major practical contribution was to rally small disparate groups of British osteopaths chiropractors and naturopaths into some cohesion, with himself at the helm of his BSO. From within the IAO under J Martin Littlejohn's tutelage, British Osteopathy evolved, independent of the

AOA and its associated British wing the BOA, to eventually prosper and expand decades later throughout Europe and the Antipodes.

Thus the developments in Littlejohn's career in the USA and the colleagues he encountered therein were the cause of his thoughts and actions, the effect of which was to be seen on this side of the Atlantic. A T Still's death in 1917 accelerated a minority reforming cohort of American osteopathic physicians to admonish the predominant traditionalist view. Impatient for tangible evidence of the existence of the osteopathic spinal lesion and its effect as a major causation of illness and disease, it intensified its cause for the integration of the materia medica syllabus within all osteopathic schools. Still's traditionalist supporters were being harried in the Midwest states, their classical heartland, by a vibrant, dynamic chiropractic profession. By contrast the reformers were being pursued on the other flank by their medical antagonists endeavouring to obstruct their ambition for full state licence to practice as physicians and surgeons.[53] The lines were indeed set for success by reformers, not only to implement materia medica against the wishes of the traditionalists, but also for a Flexner-type reformation of all schools, to confound the American Medical Association. Although J Martin Littlejohn had postulated a third way, it no longer seemed relevant as changes towards instituting a medical curriculum came into effect. If only Littlejohn had promoted and defended more robustly his Chicago inspired ideas twenty five years beforehand, based on a clear simple hypothesis, (namely that an individual unable to adjust or adapt to events can suffer general health dysfunction), then events might have turned out differently.

The mid 1930s became a crossroads for osteopathy on both sides of the Atlantic, yet it has always faced problems of direction, ever since its inception 125 years ago. In Britain, Littlejohn brooded over his poor relationship with Streeter and his enmity with BOA colleagues. No one contemplated what cataclysm would be wrought when the imminence of a Bill to regulate osteopaths would enter its House of Lords select committee stage. Whereas the osteopathic profession represented by the ODL, BOA BSO and its alumnal IAO were disunited, disorganised, uncoordinated and amateurish, the medical opposition, in contrast, were professional, well researched, strategically prepared and ruthless. A metaphorical tsunami would occur, which would take UK osteopathy almost six decades to recover from.

1. Hall T E *The Contribution of John Martin Littlejohn to Osteopathy* The Osteopathic Publishing Company 1952 pp. 15-16
2. Collins M. *Osteopathy in Britain: The First hundred years* Booksurge 2005 pp.11-12
3. There are many documents showing all three (JML, brothers James and David) using FSSc from Kirksville and in the prospectuses of the Chicago College up to and including 1902-1912. We do not know whether James and David became members or used the letters arbitrarily. Similarly, JML may well have been given some 'honorary' dispensation to use this title and since he gave lectures to this organisation on visits to London, he might have enrolled James and David too under a family membership.
4. Report from the Select Committee of the House of Lords, Select Committee of the. *Registration and Regulation of Osteopaths Bill*. London: H.M. Stationery Office, 1935: 3510-3511.
5. Ibid : 3503-3510.; T E Hall end note 30 p.42
6. There is mention of a scientific society meeting in Upper Norwood up to 1894 whether this is the same Society for Science, Letters & Arts is another matter. (*The Norwood Author- Arthur Conan Doyle & The Norwood Years (1891-194)* by Alastair Duncan ISBN 978-1-904312-69-7). Crystal Palace did become a London suburb, in 1890s onwards Upper Norwood might well have been named de facto, Crystal Palace by its residents. The building itself was burned down in 1936.
7. Museum of Osteopathic Medicine, A T Still University, Kirksville, Mo. USA. C.E. Still letter to Dr Ernest Roberts, Harrogate, Yorkshire, England 23-03-1900.
8. NOA. Scanned material. Further J M Littlejohn further documents. Waring G.P. *History of Dunham Medical School*. Edited by W H King *The History of Homeopathy and Its Institutions in America* . The Lewis Publishing Co. New York and Chicago. 1905 Volume III. Chapter 3. p. 6.
9. *Journal of the Science of Osteopathy* 1902 p.52 JM Littlejohn was a contributor, could he have written this?
10. Collins M. p.12
11. Sands L, archivist at BMA, could not substantiate this claim 22-04-2012.
12. Forlow, D. Local historian in Lake Bluff, correspondence by email 19-07-2012. (copies held in NOA.J Martin Littlejohn archive)
13. James, the eldest, was an Ear, Nose, and Throat Consultant and a Director on the BSO Board of management for many years; Edgar and John, both qualified at the BSO, Edgar was briefly vice-Dean but gave up the profession, opening a bicycle shop in Benfleet, Essex but died in World War II in India; John continued in the profession but was disinclined to take part in professional matters.
14. Hall T E p. 31
15. ibid pp.30-31
16. ibid ppp.32-33
17. NOA. Scanned material. J Martin Littlejohn archive. JM Littlejohn family and sundries. JML's Family Tree p.2
18. Forlow, D Email 27-08-2012 (copies held in NOA.J Martin Littlejohn archive)
19. Collins, M. p.44
20. NOA. Scanned material. BOA documents. 1915 British Osteopathic Society membership and undated British Osteopathic Association membership.
21. Collins M p.16-17
22. Inglis, B. Book Club Associates. Glasgow1980 *Natural Medicine*. p. 69.
23. Medical Officers of Health to the parliamentary Report as to the Practice of Medicine and Surgery by unqualified Persons in the United Kingdom (1910) .
24. Collins, p.8.
25. Barker H A, *Leaves from My Life* Hutchinson & Co London 1927 p.124
26. British Osteopathic Association *"Osteopathy in Wartime."* (1943) p.5.
27. Booth, E.R. *History of Osteopathy* Caxton Press Cincinnati 1924 p.652.

28 NOA.Scanned material. BOA. British Osteopathic Society 1915 directory
29 NOA LCOM/Miscellaneous/File 1 *Speech by Noel Buxton MP* House of Commons 14th August 1917 pp.1-3.
30 British Osteopathic Association *"Osteopathy in Wartime."* (1943). pp.15-16.
31 BMA medico-political committee minutes June 6 1917 p.683. Item 120.
32 Inglis, Natural Medicine. p.73-4.
33 Collins, p.49
34 British School of Osteopathy *Prospectus 1927-8.*
35 Collins M. pp. 15-19
36 MacDonald K. *Osteopathy and the its Position in the British Isles* Reprint of lecture in the House of Commons, Tuesday 31 March 1925. pp. 1-20.
37 BSO *Prospectus* 1924-5 pp.4-5
38 Kennard A and S: interview DVD 2011.
39 BSO *Prospectus* 1927-8
40 BSO *Prospectus* 1927-8
41 Osteopathic Association Clinic (OAC) opened by George Bernard Shaw 1927 National Osteopathic Archive (NOA), London LCOM File Box 1 early documents code: NOA/LCOM/ early/ file box 1/0304
42 NOA, IAO council meetings 1925-1942 Vol. I pp17-19, 21
43 Ibid. p.25
44 Letters from J M Littlejohn to Trenear Michell DO 1933-5 : National Osteopathic Archive. J Martin Littlejohn Archive File box 1 (code: NOA/JML/filebox1/0104)
45 Pheils, M.T. (1994) "Thank you Mr Shaw" *British Medical Journal* 309 (6920): 1724-1726.
46 Canning J. *Osteopathy a Basic Science* John Martin Littlejohn Memorial Lecture 1956 pp.4-9
47 Littlejohn J M *Personal writings and Letters* NOA. J M Littlejohn Archive p.1
48 Streeter W A *The New Healing.* Methuen & Co London 1932 pp. 138-140
49 ibid pp.2-3
50 Littlejohn J M NOA. *Personal writings and Letters* p.4
51 ibid p.5
52 ibid pp 6-9
53 BMA 'Quality of Osteopathic Education in the USA' *BMA Committee on Osteopathy Part 4* no. Ost.17 1 February 1935 pp.6-7

Chapter 5

The House of Lords Select Committee Hearing 1935

The early 1930s saw a culmination of J Martin Littlejohn's dedication to his British School of Osteopathy (BSO). No one knew more than him the fragility of this decade-old institution: the school carried out the successful graduation of more than 40 students[1] but it was heavily financially dependent on him, and he was also responsible for a sizeable number of student loans.[2]

His daily routine, although mentioned in the previous chapter, needs reiterating. It was punishing. Rising at 6.30am he boarded the London train to make a 35 mile journey to his rooms in Dover Street in order to practice from 9.00am until around 2.30pm. He would then walk across Green Park to arrive at the BSO, 16 Buckingham Gate, for lectures starting at 3.00pm through until 6.00pm. Lectures over, he spent the next couple of hours until after 8.00pm writing innumerable correspondence to all and sundry in his BSO office. Legend has it that the Littlejohn family used the top floor as its London residence. However, other sources suggest that he would head for home in Essex, a pressing routine for any man, especially one in his 60s.[3]

On that train journey returning to Badger Hall he might well have reflected with satisfaction how he had guided his BSO through some vitriolic periods. Only eight years before he had turned down the British Osteopathic Association's attempt to take over his school. He could reminisce how it survived the BOA's dismissal of all contact and his reaction to resign as BOA president and his BOA membership too. From this shaky beginning the BSO became a beacon of learning for an amorphous group of individualistic British trained osteopaths. It embraced students from the North and West of England from defunct schools and their alumnal associations. Whereas the BOA was centred round London and the home counties, in contrast the BSO alumni and its association was demographically more evenly spread.

JML would have thought little about how these groups had been assimilated with scant regard for academic rigour. Instead their infectious enthusiasm for osteopathy and allegiance to him was profound compensation. Furthermore he could look on with family pride to see that Edgar, his second son, was BSO vice-Dean and taking a vital part in assisting his father.[4] JML's resoluteness and forthright endeavour to maintain a British trained osteopathic enclave, regardless of its American roots, must have given him satisfaction, especially considering that the school's numbers were fast approaching those of the BOA membership. He refuted another BOA attempt to obtain a Royal Charter in 1931[5] and two years later Dr Mellor, an ardent BOA member, had to admit,

> 'The BOA could never benefit from contact with the BSO, that equally Osteopathy could not obtain recognition so long as everyone was obliged to go over to the USA to obtain a diploma. It was, therefore, very probable that a Bill would be passed by the medical men to limit osteopaths in their work or to bring manipulation into medicine. It was agreed....to build up the (BOA) clinic.'[6]

JML was totally aware of this essential gridlock even though some superficial rapprochement of relations had taken place to enable Bob Boothby MP to introduce his private members' bill, which had been sponsored by Wilfrid Streeter's lay supported Osteopathic Defence League (ODL).[7]

Streeter ploughed on with his influential society supporters, determined to address the state registration and regulation of osteopaths, though this last effort failed too. He tried to convince the BOA and Littlejohn's BSO and its association, Incorporated Association of Osteopaths (IAO), to drop all mutual hostilities and reservations to produce a unified coherent policy towards this legislative end. However, suspicion and mistrust pervaded all three groups and therefore ensured that any advance in legislative procedures through parliament were essentially bound to fail. In 1931, Streeter's Osteopathic Defence League found sufficient favour with W M Adamson MP for him to introduce a private members bill to establish a new osteopaths' board to regulate osteopathy in Britain and register all trained osteopaths. Meanwhile the BOA, intent on protecting its own interests, tried to renegotiate terms to the advantage of its own members. They demanded majority representation on the new board and similar rights as the medical profession to issue birth and death certificates.[8]

Whether the BOA plan was to scupper Streeter's efforts or simply a naïve act to elevate its members on a par with their medical counterparts, the bill failed to arouse any parliamentary interest.⁹ This may have been precisely the BOA intention so as to demote any efforts made by the ODL, whilst pursuing other self-serving causes.

Sure enough, the BOA had petitioned again for a Royal Charter providing them exclusive rights to the title Osteopath and exclusive ownership of the title, "Registered Osteopath (RO)". Its parliamentary ally Arthur Greenwood MP had arranged an interview with Lord Palmer, President of the Privy Council, to allay any fears of the BOA wishing to create alarm and despondency among allied groups. But Palmer was not assuaged by Greenwood. More tellingly he replied that there was much opposition to this Charter. Greenwood then attempted to placate medical opposition by requesting a meeting of those Privy Councilors of its medical committee to counter any medical establishment opposition of their intentions. Furthermore, Greenwood continued to explain that the BOA did not wish to increase its members' medical rights but only to protect the word "osteopath" from unqualified practitioners. Nevertheless, the Privy Council threw out its proposals citing not only opposition from the medical profession but also from their own supposed osteopathic allies: ODL, BSO and IAO.[10]

During this time JML complained of being ignored and excluded from any of the legislative and Privy Council proposals in favour of osteopathic advancement made by Streeter or BOA representatives. Even though they needed his support as BSO Dean and that of its alumnal association. Streeter's ODL and BOA self-seeking activities were viewed with considerable disdain by Littlejohn.[11] Moreover Sir Herbert Barker, once an esteemed Streeter ally, was showing signs of ambivalence by distancing himself from osteopathic aspirations, while a repentant medical profession began offering its own belated respect for his bonesetting skills.

Littlejohn and Barker appeared to get on together for some time. Barker had been duly appointed a BSO director of the school board. He in turn probably recommended the BSO to his nephews, Vivian and George Barrow, who both graduated, George becoming a BSO trustee by 1935.[12] It was James Mennell, an orthopaedic consultant at St. Thomas's Hospital London, (an institution with reasonably longstanding manipulative traditions) who extolled the virtues of all manipulators and cited the medical profession as " warped with prejudice by claims made and dismissive of the story told by patients, with a sneer".[13]

Thus grew Barker's own individual reputation resulting in *The Times* praising his skills and urging the medical profession to amend past grievances against him.[14] Moreover, invitations to demonstrate his techniques to a medical audience were being sought. Meanwhile Streeter warned his old friend and supporter not to waver and accept token acknowledgement from medical people: "make an offer to demonstrate your methods as a *quid pro quo* for recognition".[15] However Barker was warming to these more positive medical soundings and Streeter's fears were realised only too soon. It became part of British Medical Association (BMA) policy to separate people such as Barker and Kelman MacDonald, consultant physician cum osteopath, from the general run-of the-mill bonesetter and osteopath.[16] Furthermore it hardly helped the osteopathic cause when Barker's letter in *The Times* explained essential differences in approach and ethos between Bonesetting methods and Osteopathic procedures.[17]

Meanwhile another futile attempt by Streeter and his ODL to proceed towards statutory regulation was made by Bob Boothby MP in 1933. This time at least none of the osteopathic quartet appeared to thwart its private members' announcement, but the motion singularly failed to produce any momentum in the Commons. Moreover, the BOA membership had begun to comprehend its paradoxical situation: neither could it countenance the BSO as an osteopathic training establishment, nor could a British Minister of Health sanction any group whose training exclusively took place in a foreign land, that being the USA. The BOA was caught between a rock and a hard place.[18] But the indefatigable Streeter was not to be deterred. By 1934 the House of Commons had approved the first reading of an Osteopaths Bill and sent it to a select committee of the House of Lords for enquiry.

Whilst the assorted osteopathic groups patched up their differences through compromise, they still could not work out any preparative plan of strategy, action and consequence, either individually or as a group, nor delineate different areas of responsibility. Meanwhile medical authorities opposed to the Osteopaths Bill met up to focus on their own specific areas of expertise. BMA and Royal Colleges would carry out strategic planning: the BMA would focus on osteopathic credentials, political aspirations and theory; the Royal Colleges would examine osteopathic scientific criteria; and the General Medical Council would study osteopathic professionalisation. The BMA Committee opposed to an Osteopaths Bill met for the first time on 4th June 1934.[19]

This committee met regularly to prepare as detailed a case as possible opposing statutory regulation of osteopaths. The team composed of BMA's medical secretary, George Anderson, its assistant secretary, Charles Hill, better known as "the Radio Doctor" for his BBC broadcast contributions, and Dr C O Hawthorne. Anderson and Hill were given the majority of responsibility to research osteopathy, whilst Hawthorne focused on osteopathic diagnosis and treatment. It became apparent fairly quickly that their purpose was not to substantiate their views concerning osteopathic validity and effectiveness but for the osteopathic profession to provide evidence of proof. Although the osteopathic lesion as a major factor in causing disease was considered by them to be highly spurious, some agreement was accepted that a biophysical component of local effects appeared reasonable.[20] The BMA team relied heavily on help from The American Medical Association (AMA). They drew on the AMA's own experience of decades opposing state legislation giving osteopathic practitioners full licences to practice on a par with American physicians and surgeons.

An AMA report outlined a struggle between Osteopaths and a more vibrant Chiropractors, illustrating remarkable similarities between pioneering osteopathy and present day chiropractic. Furthermore it dramatically highlighted a split in the osteopathic movement between those who wished to continue along traditional practice as emulated by its founder Andrew Taylor Still, and those mainly collegiate entry graduates emerging as a cohort of clinically more discerning practitioners with full medical licence to practice. The report concluded with a prediction of the imminent demise of osteopathy and an irresistible decline in chiropractic too.[21] Over time papers were presented and discussed at BMA committee meetings on the strengths and weaknesses of osteopathy. The BMA team could have been congratulated in preparing a well researched dossier to hand to its solicitor, Oswald A Hempson.

It was all well and good to produce documents opposing osteopathy but Hempson's strategy was to introduce into a House of Lords select committee a judicial court atmosphere with osteopathic representatives being the accused and medical opposition as prosecuting counsel. Hempson's policy was to feed his counsel with material to divide three of the four osteopathic personalities, knowing their well-known animosity towards one another. Their cooperation during the Bill's passage through parliament was a thin veneer, masquerading as a united front.[22] Moreover, Kelman MacDonald was osteopathy's strongest witness, so it would be the objective of BMA counsel to separate him from the others by emphasising his superior medical qualifications. If only all osteopaths obtained MacDonald's medical attainments then there would be no reason to place such a Bill before parliament? Counsel would persevere to drive a wedge between the BOA's representative MacDonald and Littlejohn's BSO as an inadequate training establishment and also osteopathy's understanding of disease causation which differed from MacDonald's own view which was much more orthodox.[23]

Tactics would be utilised to show the apparent differences in MacDonald's worthy credentials and perceptions compared with Streeter, Littlejohn and Ray Harvey Foote, American colleague and JML's friend and confidant. Overriding priority was made to cast the BSO as a fraudulent school and Littlejohn as the instigator of the fraud by awarding diplomas based on a four years' curriculum when students had never completed such a course. The BMA dossier on Littlejohn provides evidence of this and other misdemeanours and how both Littlejohn and the BSO were considered the main weakness to exploit during the hearing.[24] Even though Hempson had little time for Streeter's 'abysmal ignorance', it is MacDonald's acknowledged superior class versus his osteopathic colleagues' lower attainments which would be pursued by BMA counsels, steered by Hempson in the background.[25] The BMA choice of chief and assistant counsel was critically important not only to defeat the Bill during the select committee stage but also to prevent in the future a parliamentary motion and any further argument of any eccentric individual or cult posing a threat to the medical establishment by introducing a training course analogous to medicine whilst proposing outlandish fantasy.[26] Hempson supported the gifted Wilfred Green KC as senior counsel and Hal Dickens as his junior but there was a problem, Wilfred Green had already been retained by the Royal Colleges. Alternatively, Sir William Jowitt KC was considered an effective alternative and was instructed to represent the BMA.[27] Everything was now set in place for the inaugural meeting of the select committee of the House of Lords: Osteopaths Bill on Monday 4 March 1935.

Ii was a bleak, grey, late winter morning at 11.00am when the select committee met in a compact room with lofty windows, looking out on the river Thames. It was agreed that the committee would meet every Monday and Friday, with midweek and weekend recess. It comprised of seven members, including Lord Elibank, who was for the Bill and Lord Dawson of Penn, a distinguished medical man, opposing. They sat

Chapter 5

around a large mahogany table, while facing the table was a retinue of imposing counsel representing the various proposing and opposing groups. Sir William Jowitt, BMA senior counsel, was tall and genial in appearance and his opposite number, J H Thorpe, senior counsel for the osteopathic parties, was noted as being lanky and good-looking. Somehow, sandwiched further along, in cramped space, were three rows of interested observers. The general atmosphere seemed impartial and matters evenly paced as the meeting unfolded. After the usual introductory statements Wilfrid Streeter, representing the Osteopathic Defence League, was called as the first witness. [28]

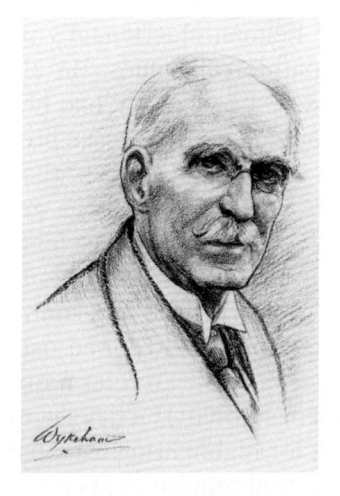

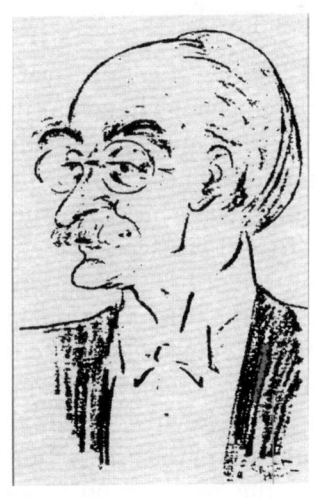

JML fondly portrayed by BSO colleagues

79

Streeter appeared over three sessions of the enquiry, and interestingly there was a complete contrast of views on his performance over these three days. He was questioned on his finger technique by Lord Dawson, robustly performed in Ear, Nose and Throat conditions. Hempson writes to Jowitt during the first recess that the select committee gives his BMA client an ideal opportunity for Jowitt to nail the "fallacious nature of osteopathy....... and put this matter at rest once and for all".

Hempson's correspondence starts by presenting the 'low-down' on Kelman MacDonald, J Martin Littlejohn and Harvey-Foote, the remaining principal osteopathic witnesses.[29] He urges Jowitt to compare the superior quality of Kelman MacDonald's training as a consultant physician to his osteopathic colleagues. He also writes that he was not convinced that the select committee had been made fully aware of Streeter's ignorance of anatomy, and disease processes.[30] On the second day, Streeter's ally Mrs Chesterton reports that Jowitt's strategy was to pitch questioning on a scientific basis as an argument against the validity of osteopathy versus orthodox scientific medicine. Streeter struggled in this part of procedure, doing his best to veer away from scientific explanations, preferring the less controversial topic of public policy of statutory regulation of all trained osteopaths. However, Mrs Chesterton acknowledges that "Mr Streeter more than held his own but to the lay-mind Sir William's (Jowitt) tactics seemed feeble".[31] By contrast Hempson praises Jowitt for highlighting osteopathic training standards to be similar to basic medical requirements rather than based on quasi-scientific 'sectarian' principles.

During the next part of the investigation, over four decisive sessions, the atmosphere appeared to change in favour of the Bill. Hempson in a letter to George Anderson, BMA medical secretary, admits that allowing, at the last minute, grateful patients to extol the virtues of osteopathic treatment to their Lordships, was a big error, one that should be desisted by Jowitt from then on. He criticises Jowitt for becoming "bogged down in scientific and pseudo-scientific explanations" and presses him to keep to the salient point, comparing MacDonald's provenance to other osteopaths.[32] Furthermore, Hempson writes to Hal Dickens, BMA junior counsel, about BMA officials showing "profound dissatisfaction at the perfunctory manner in which Jowitt is dealing with this case, and the way in which the point of view of the association (BMA) has either been ignored, or relegated to the background".[33] An osteopathic onlooker states, "from the opening of the enquiry beginning with Mr Streeter's evidence, through eager and unsolicited patients, there was a crescendo of interest, a gathering momentum of belief in the osteopathic cause that reached its climax with the testimony of Dr Kelman MacDonald. The general feeling was not only that the necessity for the Bill had been completely demonstrated but that, for the first time, the amazing possibilities of the new healing (osteopathy) had been shown".[34]

Meanwhile, further news (kept in confidence by Anderson and Hempson) contained information that a Mary Maxwell had been treated osteopathically by MacDonald the day before his final hearing and had been found dead in bed, the following morning, 22 March 1935.[35] Would they use this new evidence to try to sully MacDonald's reputation? However, Hempson and the team had other things to use with considerable effect - the quality and existence of BSO instruction in the basic medical subjects of anatomy and physiology, "The whole thing is a fraud from beginning to end".[36] Or as an osteopathic observer put it, "And then came the Littlejohn *debacle*".[37] (her italics).

From a detailed four page memorandum, the BMA strategy against J Martin Littlejohn was drawn up by Hempson, the BMA's solicitor and Charles Hill, BMA assistant medical secretary. They would make certain that JML, his school, his association with William Looker and his Manchester school alumni would be heavily criticized, and that British Osteopathy would be damaged irreparably.[38] One has to reiterate that the BMA deployed various tactics: overwhelming research against the Bill, strategies of a personal, academic and professional nature to denigrate all four potential osteopathic witnesses, and exploitation of osteopathy's disunity, ill-conceived explanations and naïve concepts. Littlejohn must have had grave misgivings about attending and participating in the whole process when, during the select committee session of Friday 22 March 1935, he took the stand, following an extensive and confident performance by MacDonald.

Harold Murphy, junior counsel for the osteopathic bodies, outlined Littlejohn's academic credentials, his connections with osteopathic education and, specifically, his role at the BSO's helm. There was an adjournment in his evidence to call further lay-witnesses.[39] Subsequently, Murphy recalled Littlejohn to confirm further aspects of the BSO, its curriculum and staffing. Hovering over these niceties was the presence of Sir William Jowitt, somewhat straining at the leash, after Hempson's remonstration about his previous ineffectual performances during the hearing.[40] Soon Jowitt was able to demonstrate his courtroom prowess by launching into Littlejohn's many academic credentials, dissecting their provenance and causing those present to doubt Littlejohn's intellectual integrity and his ability to answer Jowitt's challenges with any clarity or confidence.[41] During his cross-questioning Jowitt painted a disparaging and shifty picture of Littlejohn, who fared badly, shell-shocked by the personal nature of these attacks. Fortunately for JML, a week-end interposed between this and the next select committee session, which allowed him and the osteopathic legal team time to regroup. It was unfortunate for Jowitt who sensed that he not only had Littlejohn on the metaphorical ropes but the whole case for an Osteopaths Bill was now in dire straits.

When Monday came, Littlejohn's attitude as an obviously unwilling witness predominated his answers, and his diffidence, hesitations and bewilderment remained. Unfortunately his resultant monosyllabic responses to Jowitt's questioning and jibes came over badly to those in the room. Far from helping osteopathy's case, JML came across as a grudging unhelpful presence, which played even more unwittingly into his opponents' hands. Further Jowitt taunts produced even more hesitancy and shuffling, adding to his poor disposition.[42]

As Mrs Chesterton, an osteopathic sympathizer, wrote, "It was a deplorable performance.....his failure to recall important facts did not help the case. Indeed as time went on, I realised his evidence must have had an unfortunate influence on the issue for the last part of his cross-examination was far worse than the first. It was after his disingenuous opening that I felt a change of atmosphere among the obviously lay members of the public present. The keenness of their interest had flattened. The virtue seemed to go out of the matter; and there was a general sense of depression which increased as the interrogation went on."[43]

Under such examination and scrutiny, JML's reputation, diligence as BSO dean and the BSO's competency as a training establishment were disassembled piece by piece. Osteopathy as a healing therapy, its diagnosis with the osteopathic lesion as its rationale, and manipulative treatment, were thoroughly discredited.[44]

Mrs Chesterton's continued attendance and reporting encapsulated the session, and her words describing events have a ring of truth, "Looker students and graduates were granted a BSO diploma after one year's work. They were sent eight exam papers to their respective homes with every opportunity of looking up the answers........Sir William Jowitt demonstrated how discreditable and how irregular this act".[45] For a large part of the day Littlejohn had succumbed to intense hostile interrogation by counsel. He characterised the ineptness of poor preparation and lack of respectful teamwork among the diverse osteopathic groups. He was perceived as the weakest and most vulnerable witness to fall victim under interrogation and he duly paid the price. His academic laxity collecting various dubious academic awards, and tolerance of inadequate training standards and facilities, rebounded in a most telling way. As Mrs Chesterton remonstrated, "I have no wish to do Dr Littlejohn any injustice, and for this reason, I put this view on record. For myself, I can only speak as to the impression left upon me by his evidence.......But, to my mind, his admission settled the issue. Dr Littlejohn had defeated the Bill".[46]

To all intents and purposes she was correct in her opinion. Moreover, at the next session on Friday 29 March 1935, Sir William Jowitt drove home the BMA opposition of not countenancing an Osteopaths Bill of any description. Over the next four working days of the select committee, the full force majeure of august members of the medical and scientific professions reasoned against and unraveled systematically a case for promoting such a Bill.[47] Additionally, this sustained attack was planned to negate once and for all any similar group outside orthodox medicine from applying for statutory regulation, based on unscientific principles but utilising a medical curriculum to foster its intentions.[48]

One particular person played a critical part in opposing the Bill with his constant attendance on the selection committee panel, namely Lord Dawson of Penn, especially his interchange with MacDonald, Streeter and most tellingly, Littlejohn. [49]

Lord Dawson, soon to be elevated to Viscount, was a rare physician of the age. He trained at University College, London (UCL), (at the time perhaps the most enlightened scientific medical school in Britain), and later attained his higher MD at the London Hospital. He became an outstanding practitioner and medical politician, being appointed royal physician to both Edward VII and George V. He had wide ranging views stretching from the state of fitness of army personnel to euthanasia. This latter subject lead to his opinion that it should be carried out by the medical profession and definitely not through the process of voluntary euthanasia by lay people. Dawson's standard medical ethos, 'Doctor knows best', influenced his sentiments of maintaining medical hegemony over professional interests on health and disease by opposing such matters as the osteopathic statutory regulation through parliament.[50]

On 12th April 1935, following private discussions between MacDonald, Lord Elibank and the pro-campaigners' legal team, Thorpe and Murphy called a halt to select committee proceedings. Thorpe read out a statement that the four osteopathic bodies no longer wished to continue with the Bill.[51] The inevitability and withdrawal of the Bill provided medical institutions with a decisive victory and thorough vindication for preparing such a well researched and professionally coordinated campaign. Littlejohn and Osteopathy had been trounced by forthright planning, legal heavy weights and clever medical opponents whose own methods of treatment were not wholly based on science either. The ultimate message to any group within alternative or pseudo religious medical circles, willing to take on the medical establishment, was beware! This defeat in the select committee "trial" demonstrated the opinions of the time and challenged any from attempting to do the same in the future.

There was to be no sympathetic consideration for Littlejohn, nor for his role as BSO dean when the report was published on 17th July 1935. It was a stark statement of fact by the Select committee, reminding all of those two days, 22nd and 25th March 1935, "The only existing establishment in this country for the education and examining of osteopaths was exposed in the course of evidence before us, as being of negligible importance, inefficient for its purpose and above all, in thoroughly dishonest hands".[52]

The next part of Littlejohn's life was taken up with the defence of his reputation, his beloved school and the failing power to cope with his intensive weekly routine. Undoubtedly he was cherished by his family, friends, his faculty, students and patients, but there is no hiding from the fact that osteopathy, not for the first time and certainly not the last, became even more defensive, inward looking and at a proverbial cross-roads of where to go, for the foreseeable future.

---

1   NOA.Scanned Material. BSO Early Documents. JML BSO 1929
2   Canning, James *Osteopathy a Basic Science* London: Board of Governors BSO. 1956. pp. 7-10.
    There is some difference whether he started lecturing at 2.00pm or 3.00pm.

Chapter 5

3 NOA Scanned Material. J Martin Littlejohn Archive. Littlejohn Further Documents. House of Lords Dinner 2nd March 1934.
4 NOA/CIDove/Filebox3/0102 *BSO Prospectus* 1934-35 p.2
5 Streeter, W A *The New Healing* London: Methuen & Co.1932.pp.232-5
6 BOA Council minutes November 1933 p.116
7 ibid 2 May 1933 pp.104-5
8 Collins, M., *Osteopathy in Britain: the first hundred years* London: Booksurge 2005 pp56-7
9 Streeter, W.A. *The New Healing*. London: Methuen & Co. 1932. p.230
10 ibid p.232
11 Littlejohn J M *Personal writings and Letters* J M Littlejohn Archive: NOA/JML/filebox1/0104 Hand-written notes pp.1-9
12 Collins, M., p.127 & p.291
13 Streeter W.A., *The Osteopathic Bulletin* ODL No.3. October 1932. NOA.BSO archives p.1
14 Inglis, B., *Natural Medicine* London: William Collins & Sons 1979 p.94
15 Streeter W.A., *The Osteopathic Bulletin* ODL No.3.p.1
16 Well H G Preface: Clegg, C. & Hill, H.A., *What is Osteopathy?* London: J.M. Dent & Sons Ltd. 1937 p.vii
17 BMA, 'BMA legal notes drawn up on McDonald, Littlejohn and letter in *The Times* from Barker.' BMA legal team. 1935
18 BOA Council minutes 2 May 1933 & November 1933 pp.104-5; p.116
19 BMJ, 'What is Osteopathy? And BMA Committee on osteopathy appointed.' *British Medical Journal* Jan.-Jun 3861-3886. 1935. 5 January 1935. P.20.
20 Hawthorne, C O 'Osteopathy as a diagnostic and therapeutic model' *BMA Committee on Osteopathy Part 3*, no. Ost. 4. 1934 p.3
21 BMA, 'Quality of Osteopathic Education in the USA' *BMA Committee on Osteopathy Part 4* no.Ost.16 1 February 1935 pp.1-3; no. Ost. 17 1 February 1935 pp. 6-7.
22 Ray Harvey Foote dossier *BMA Committee on Osteopathy* p.1
23 Kelman MacDonald dossier *BMA Committee on Osteopathy* pp.1-3
24 J Martin Littlejohn dossier *BMA Committee on Osteopathy* pp.1-4
25 Hempson, O A letter to Sir William Jowitt: O A Hempson correspondence *BMA Archives* 7 March 1935 p.2
26 Anderson, G.: Statement of objections to the Bill: O A Hempson correspondence *BMA Archives* 21 January 1935 p.1
27 Hempson, O A letter to G. Anderson: O A Hempson correspondence *BMA Archives* 4 January 1935 p.1
28 Chesterton, C., *This Body: An Experience in Osteopathy*. London: Stanley Paul & Co 1937 pp. 105-6
29 Hempson, O A letter to G. Anderson: O A Hempson correspondence *BMA Archives* 9 March 1935 pp.1-2
30 Hempson, O A letter to Sir William Jowitt: O A Hempson correspondence *BMA Archives* 7 March 1935 pp.1-2
31 Chesterton, C., p.112
32 Hempson, O A letter to G. Anderson: O A Hempson correspondence *BMA Archives* 23 March 1935 pp.1-2
33 Hempson, O A letter to Hal Dickens: O A Hempson correspondence *BMA Archives* 23 March 1935 p.1
34 Chesterton, C., pp.138-9
35 E Sharpey-Schafer to G Anderson : O A Hempson correspondence *BMA Archives* 22 March 1935 p.1
36 Hill, C., letter to O A Hempson: O A Hempson correspondence *BMA Archives* 22 March 1935 pp.1-2

37 Chesterton, C., p.139
38 BMA: 'BMA Legal Note drawn up on J Martin Littlejohn' BMA Legal team 1935 pp.1-4
39 House of Lords Select Committee, *Registration and Regulation of Osteopaths Bill*. London: HMSO, 1935 pp.210-212
40 ibid pp.216-219
41 ibid pp.220-225
42 Chesterton, C., p.137
43 ibid p.135-6
44 House of Lords Select Committee, *Registration and Regulation of Osteopaths Bill*. pp.225-260
45 Chesterton, C., p.137
46 ibid p.138
47 House of Lords Select Committee, *Registration and Regulation of Osteopaths Bill*. pp. x-xii
48 Hill, C & Clegg, H A, *What is Osteopathy?* London: H Dent & Sons 1937 pp. x-xi
49 ibid. pp. 212-256
50 Wikipedia: *Bernard Dawson, 1st Viscount Dawson of Penn*: Early life an education. One takes issue with his training at UCL, it must have included his MB BS degrees as well as his MD post graduate course at the London Hospital p.1 . Interestingly, Damien Lewis, the actor, is a great grandson.
51 House of Lords Select Committee, *Registration and Regulation of Osteopaths Bill*. pp.437-440
52 ibid p.iv

Chapter 6
The gloaming years (1936-1947)

The extent of satisfaction of the medical profession for its triple victory was profound. Firstly, the four osteopathic bodies were forced to call a halt to all parliamentary activity seeking statutory regulation, and secondly, its damning aftermath, the report by the House of Lords select subcommittee rejected a further advance of the Osteopaths Bill through parliament. Lastly, the defeat nailed a crucial intention of the medical community, which was to prevent any other alternative and pseudo-religious medical organisations from seeking similar state regulation under the guise of an orthodox medical school curriculum. This final implication hardly created a ripple among the opponents of the Bill, but among the osteopathic bodies involved in their disastrous campaign a deeper chasm appeared overnight. The British Osteopathic Association representative Kelman MacDonald tried to parry criticism of the British School of Osteopathy and its Dean, J Martin Littlejohn during his stand as a witness in the selection committee. MacDonald could neither defend what he and others determined as substandard, nor felt entirely comfortable in his criticisms of Littlejohn's BSO stewardship and student training. His was a restrained account under blunt, well prepared questioning by the BMA's counsel, Sir William Jowitt KC. Under this barrage, MacDonald did his best to convey Littlejohn's difficulties in running the BSO, but was forced to admit its deficiencies and its inadequacies as unacceptable. Not only was this utilised to the satisfaction of opponents to the Bill but also his BOA colleagues too, who roundly condemned the BSO and its head in no uncertain manner.

Littlejohn was sustained from these slings and arrows by his BSO alumni, staff and students. Several of them had supposedly inspected his various academic awards during his vilification in the select committee and claimed, with some authority, their genuine provenance.[1] It was a naïve gesture: the certificates may have looked like credible and distinguished documents but their academic credentials were largely suspect, if not scurrilous. Moreover, Littlejohn was aware of this factor too. His response to questioning about his Doctor of Law and Doctor of Philosophy is not only evasive but economical with the truth.[2] This was further affirmed by his friend Ray Harvey Foote, who was forced by osteopathic counsel to withdraw as its fourth select committee osteopathic witness as a lost cause after Littlejohn's poor performance. Harvey Foote reported back to fellow council members of the Incorporated Association of Osteopaths (soon to change its name to Osteopathic Association of Great Britain-OAGB for short) about JML's catastrophic display.

Foote regretted not being able to rescue some of the momentum created by MacDonald and its lay supporters during the select committee sittings. He presumed his own deposition might have rectified some of the impression created during Littlejohn's "unfortunate" account. Foote sought to counter any motion at the meeting to withhold financial support from the other osteopathic bodies involved in promotion of the Bill. These were formal obligations made to Wilfrid Streeter, who had orchestrated the move for statutory regulation from the outset of their parliamentary pursuit. Streeter had founded his Osteopathic Defence League, an institution for the high and mighty of British establishment to further orchestrate these ends. He also pursued Sir Herbert Barker, the celebrated bonesetter, to this cause too. However, Streeter's contempt towards Littlejohn, the BSO and its alumni before, during and aftermath of the House of Lords select committee created a begrudging recognition among them that his demand they pay their due legal fees was felt as "regrettable, considering the treatment received".[3] However the feeling of disgruntlement was to grow among rank and file alumnal members of the BSO and its retitled, Osteopathic Association of Great Britain (OAGB), directing their ire on Sir William Jowitt's BMA counsel, his annihilation of Littlejohn, Streeter's disdain towards them and further retribution towards their BOA nemesis.

With little fuss Sir Herbert Barker relinquished his BSO directorship, and the medical profession continued to offer its esteem, almost eulogising his manipulative prowess with invitations to demonstrate his techniques to medical audiences. Medical professionals even admitted a direct relationship between bonesetting, medical practice and modern orthopaedics.[4] Even though Wilfrid Streeter was mortified by the loss of Barker as friend and supporter, and the OAGB had offered Barker an honorary life membership, there is no record of his acceptance. Losing Barker's support was not the only blow to Littlejohn either.

Chapter 6

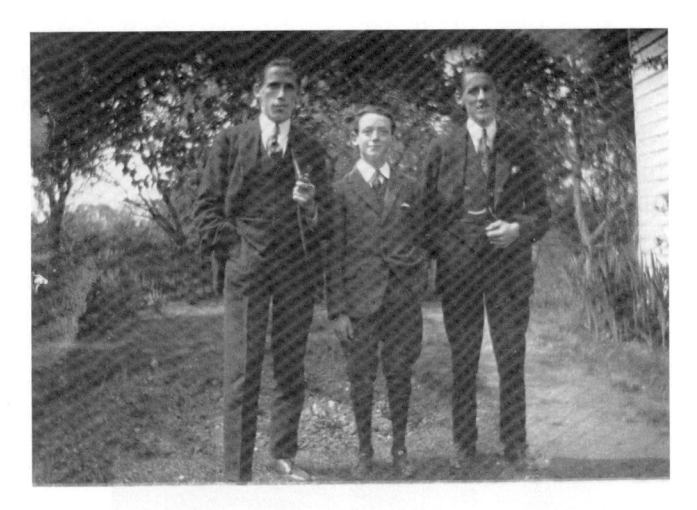

Sons: Edgar, John and James as young men

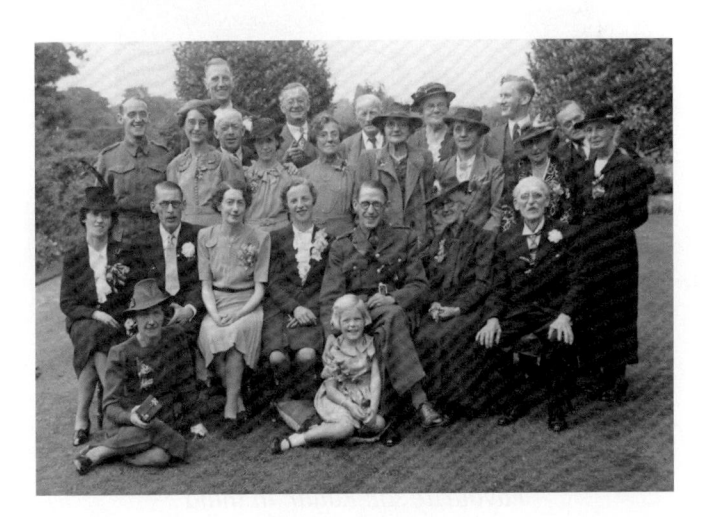

James' wedding

His son, Edgar, a BSO graduate, had been appointed vice-Dean and co-clinic superintendent at the BSO in the early 1930s. He accepted the post possibly to take pressure off his hard-working father, but Edgar clearly did not find osteopathy conducive enough and informed the family of his change of heart. Some months later, he opened a bicycle shop in Benfleet not far from the family home, Badger Hall. JML's youngest son, John, also graduated from the BSO and continued to practice until his retirement

89

in the 1960s, but shunned all opportunities to join the school faculty, administration, school board and all alumnal association posts.[5] It was left to JML's eldest son James Littlejohn to support his father through to wartime, which he did assiduously by joining the BSO board of directors, whilst taking over some of the other extraneous tasks. Even though James had gone through medical school to specialise in otorhinolaryngology, by joining the BSO board he thus allowed his father to gradually distance himself from decision making and to reduce his hectic daily routine.

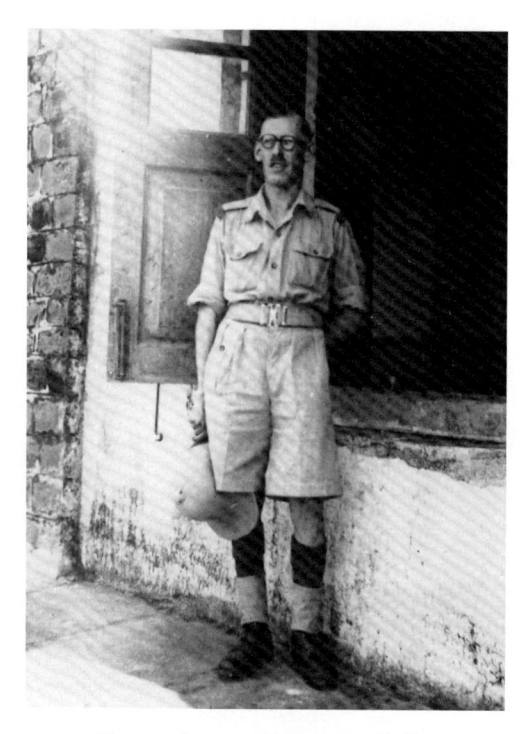

Favourite son Edgar, in India

James's extra duties came with compassion, knowing full well how his own profession had treated his father and his beloved BSO. His loyalty was undiminished during this difficult period. It allowed his father to spend much time writing articles defending himself, his school and his UK trained graduates. These were characterised by themes of Christian aspirations, criticism of the medical profession and abrasive comments about American Osteopathy.[6] More problematically, the loosening of JML's ties to the BSO left a void as to who should be appointed vice-Dean, and probably as heir and successor. Out of the ranks came a charismatic young professional musician and BSO graduate, Thomas Edward Hall.

He came to prominence within the confines of the BSO and its alumnal association, IAO, through a letter he composed for *Time and Tide* magazine, a weekly political and literary review. He penned it during a hiatus between the selection committee's conclusion and the publication of its findings. In that letter, he castigated Kelman MacDonald for his criticism of the BSO as being substandard by not training its students to a recognised attainment, and the general animosity of BOA members towards his school.[7] Without benefit of Mrs Chesterton's eyewitness account and a verbatim record, Hall's criticism of MacDonald was unfounded. During the select committee MacDonald had been targeted specifically by BMA counsel who dragged out of him, reluctantly under duress, his admittance of such critical testimonial. There was little that MacDonald could have done but limit damage. Hall's vitriol against the BOA and its members was fairer, it had been duplicitous for a decade trying to obtain advantageous precedence over their UK trained colleagues.

Tommy Hall was everything that J Martin Littlejohn was not. A physically striking presence, what the Irish call 'full of the door', he emanated confidence with his resolute Lancastrian voice. He had similar hands to the great sculptor Henry Moore, who himself loved to massage people's legs, especially females. (perhaps the softness of their skin with the delicacy of muscle and bone?) Hall was a great manipulator in the true tradition of bonesetting, but developed technical skills beyond. His forte was to embrace a thorough knowledge of anatomy with manipulative skills. One cannot envisage that this odd couple of the diminutive, studious Littlejohn and the larger-than-life Hall had too much in common, either in cerebral activity or conversation. His family perceived that JML had serious misgivings over Hall's appointment,[8] (but neither did Littlejohn possess recognised leadership qualities either). Moreover, Hall's manners were those of a character actor to be seen in Ealing Studio films: full of charm, bluster and industry. These were just the attributes to equip a young osteopath building a London West End practice, knowing his way round the various familiar watering holes but perhaps without the essential talents to steer a struggling BSO to calmer waters. However, Hall was just the person to combat any BOA derision and return it with force by rallying BSO alumni to increased invective, even bellicosity. Osteopathy's opponents must have looked on with enormous satisfaction as both sides attacked each other. Meanwhile, in the final days of the select committee, Lord Elibank and MacDonald had spoken of an alternative solution, the setting up of a voluntary register of all osteopaths.[9]

The founding of the General Council and Register of Osteopaths (GCRO) was first broached in those early days of April 1935 by Elibank, MacDonald and Streeter amidst the ashes of the Osteopaths Bill. There is little evidence that it was supported by the Minister of Health. It was osteopathic counsel who stated that a voluntary register would be formed.[10] This triumvirate was joined by Ray Harvey Foote, who had fostered membership in both associations, being US trained in an American Osteopathic Association (AOA) affiliated college, and also performing a role as a council member of the BSO alumnal Osteopathic Association of Great Britain (OAGB). Predictably, BOA officials were not persuaded by Foote to show any leniency towards Littlejohn, the BSO, OAGB, or other osteopathic groups or individuals outside their own ranks.

The GCRO was incorporated on 22 July 1936, but it would take another year for the implications of the select committee to take effect. Accordingly, there was to be retribution from BOA delegates, the details of which determined which group could become registered members. It conceded that BOA members would be accepted en bloc, and full membership was reserved for graduates of AOA affiliated schools. By contrast all BSO osteopaths and those from other establishments, home and abroad, would have to submit to a sub-category, associate membership. Their application would require an interview to prove length of service and exams to determine competency.[11] Ironically, Littlejohn must have given himself a wry smile, his records of attendance of the Kirksville course (1898-1900) for his diploma smacked of a certain casualness from various quarters: the 'P for present' box and summary of progress appears to be have been written with the same pen at one time only; and the same handwriting graced the various subjects which were taught by different persons throughout two years attendance.[12] That a Kirksville official should attempt to doctor Littlejohn's attendance on a form to fulfil his qualifications was at variance with its alumnal members joining the BOA extolling the virtues of such an institution, whilst having such a jaundiced view of Littlejohn's BSO headship and its credentials. His Kirksville osteopathic records were deemed correct for immediate approval as a full GCRO member, even though there is no record that he ever applied for membership, although John Martin Littlejohn junior definitely did so, practising with his father at the Dover Street practice.[13]

Accordingly, Littlejohn was lambasted both by counsel representing medical opponents of an Osteopaths Bill and by his BOA colleagues for certain dubious practices of awarding BSO diplomas to those with insufficient training. He had, for almost a decade, trained a cohort of UK osteopaths who would influence the outcome of osteopathic evolution for the next half century. His ways of working are disputable, but his intention to take an amorphous group of variably trained British osteopaths along a distinct evolutionary path was apocryphal. After the debacle of the select committee, Littlejohn lost the heart and spirit to maintain this avenue of entry into the profession. Others made attempts to revive this arrangement but were met by his son James, deputising for JML. Naturopathic pleas to assist in training its students were consistently acknowledged but were dealt with by a resolute negative response. Moreover, it was impossible to envisage a BOA-dominated GCRO showing equanimity to any osteopathic group looking for inclusion as full register members.

Something should be said about the BSO administration during Littlejohn's tutelage. Colin Dove (BSO principal 1968-76) suggests that all education establishments require a decent head but, most of all, an outstanding administrator: someone to organise the general functioning, maintain and coordinate staff and students' welfare, as well as retaining a grip on the finances.[14] Littlejohn was devoid of permitting anyone capable of undertaking such a task. The absence of such a person allowed osteopathy's critics to condemn BSO's inadequacies, ramshackle countenance and somewhat aimless direction. During his days as head of the Littlejohn College in Chicago, he was able to lean on a number of people for support.

In a previous chapter we discussed his brother James's ascendancy within the profession, how he developed to outclass JML in many ways, without him being quite aware of or willing to admit it.

James's medical training at Glasgow and his further postgraduate medical research in Chicago showed his professional worth. He envisaged osteopathy as an important specialisation within medicine and surgery. Indeed, he oversaw major surgery and the post surgical ward building at the Kirksville school, the completion of which so angered A T Still at its inaugural opening. From 1907 onwards he promoted the teaching of materia medica to students and its submission to the Illinois State Medical Board for college accreditation to full medical licences. Moreover, he was a very popular and gifted lecturer with some purposeful direction towards eventual full medical licences for all osteopaths. Whereas brother J Martin's foresight, however valid, was circumscribed and also, characteristically, JML found it very difficult to forgive and forget past dissensions.

Meanwhile, James was corresponding with Charlie Still in a most courteous way following the extended vendetta between the two families some five years before.[15] Furthermore, the role of Edith, James's wife, as a Littlejohn College board member and prominent among the faculty, showed she was no shrinking violet either, but played a decisive part in the college's evolution. She and James combined to steer the college in another direction from what J Martin intended, following the Flexner Report on medical education. J Martin never appeared to be aware of the rise of his brother, his political awareness in committing osteopathic medicine towards orthodoxy, the professional determination of Edith in supporting her husband, and his colleagues' collective support for James to lead the Littlejohn College, and its metamorphosis into the Chicago College of Osteopathy, headed by Carl McConnell with James as his deputy.

J Martin's son, James, an ENT consultant, might have had some sympathy for his uncle's orthodox medical aspirations too. However, his father and uncle never communicated again.[16] Be that as it may, there were others to defend J Martin's reputation and his BSO.

By midsummer 1937 the General Council and Register of Osteopaths (GCRO) was set up to admit en bloc the first cohort of 22 BOA members (which consisted of about 25% of the total BOA membership), thus not a clarion call for total commitment to this new institution. However, they were permitted five representatives on the GCRO council, which was five more than any other osteopathic group. This BOA quintet would "govern all their future activities and determine their status". Resentful of this was a vociferous OAGB faction led by T E Hall who railed at the injustice of having to undergo individual applications for membership. Only a specified entry as associate member was allowed, outrageously, with no voting rights and no representation on the GCRO Council either and finally, no BSO accreditation to boot.[17]

Subsequently another cohort of GCRO members would be admitted at the end of the year - a smaller contingent of 15 US AOA affiliated trained BOA osteopaths applied en bloc. It dawned on MacDonald, Elibank, and Streeter that not all BOA members could be enticed to join. A number thought that the GCRO was superfluous to their needs and that the BOA did a more than reasonable job in providing sufficient, adequate professional services. MacDonald's team soon realised that the GCRO would become a farcical institution, containing a rump of BOA full members and vestigial assortment of non-voting associates. There had to be an alternative solution to ease entry for BSO graduates as full members and some chance of BSO accreditation. GCRO officials turned to Harvey Foote for help.[18]

During discussions MacDonald and Streeter outlined Harvey Foote's crucial mediation role as a US AOA affiliated trained osteopath, his position as OAGB Council member, BSO Board member and friend of J Martin Littlejohn. A further plan was hatched by the trio for MacDonald and Streeter to placate BOA opposition preventing full rights admission en bloc of OAGB members, while Harvey Foote would advise the OAGB council against a subsequent boycott of the GCRO. He suggested that three council members comprising of senior officials, Milne, Van Straten and Saul, should individually apply for admittance. Once this happened these three new full GCRO members would advocate for en bloc OAGB/BSO consideration.[19]

Muddying the waters further was the status of members of the National Society of Osteopaths, naturopathic osteopaths and an assortment of individuals, the very people that Littlejohn would have welcomed as prospective BSO candidates for supplementary training a decade before. After the House of Lords report this was no longer considered possible. Unfortunately, in early August 1937, Ray Harvey Foote died, aged 57. He had laid down a formula by which BSO graduates could join the GCRO as full members with reasonable dignity. J Martin Littlejohn extolled Foote's virtues in an eulogy a month later, praising him as an unsung hero for ten years who gave succour to his UK trained colleagues and supported Littlejohn and his BSO since the break with the BOA, whilst retaining contacts with his BOA colleagues.[20] Once the senior OAGB officials Milne, Van Straten and Saul had been accepted as full members they were able to promote full GCRO rights to OAGB members.

Meanwhile T Edward Hall in his role as BSO vice-Dean and President of the OAGB was showing no signs of any compromise towards the GCRO's extended olive branch. Hall was supported throughout this campaign of

GCRO boycott by his capable wife, Dorothy Wood, a medical practitioner. Throughout their time together Hall and Wood formed a formidable partnership, engaging in money raising activities, but also raising funds personally towards a BSO X-ray department, founding a BSO gynaecological department, and providing the Dorothy Wood Gold Medal for the top BSO student in their final year at a time when very few medical doctors would have much sympathy towards osteopathy.[21] In a sense, J Martin Littlejohn was appreciative of Dorothy Wood's commitment to the BSO, running a department and donating annual prizes to students, besides supporting her husband's collegiate ambitions and Hall's own technical wizardry as a gifted manipulator. Significantly Hall remained adamant that there would be no en bloc admittance of OAGB members supporting his register boycott until the GCRO had accredited the BSO. Whether it was Harvey Foote's legacy or MacDonald's magisterial powers plus the three OAGB officials' gifts of persuasion, we don't know, but thirty OAGB/BSO graduates ignored Hall's plea, plus six further BOA members, all attaining full GCRO membership in June 1938. The disparity between the two groups was down to 10, giving BOA a useful majority. Moreover, by the end of the year, the difference was one, with eleven new BSO and two BOA entrees. Consequently, BSO graduate formal representation on the GCRO council appeared and increased with each incremental intake.

The next crucial event to take place was a GCRO inspection of the BSO and its dependence on a majority Littlejohn share holding, two decisive steps before accreditation.[22]

Why did Littlejohn decide to transfer his BSO shares to an independent Board of Trustees, when he had obstinately refused to do so a decade before? Firstly, any prior negotiations depended upon a favourable outcome from the inspection team made up of BOA members. Although eventual accreditation was given to the BSO with a number of BOA members joining the school faculty, many felt uncomfortable over this decision. Especially those BOA members who never forgave Littlejohn's disrepute nor the modest educational standards at the BSO. However, Littlejohn, with some diffidence, after its early patronising attitude towards the BSO alumni, entered into talks with GCRO officials to hand over BSO control and sale of assets.

With his solicitor's help, Littlejohn negotiated a £240 settlement, (more than an average annual salary) for his 80% shares. The process was long-drawn. Over and above this, the BSO had become a burden not only to him but his family as well. Many BSO students had been reliant on JML from its inception, by delaying the payment of their school fees to the extent that the Littlejohn family acted as a private bank. In order to compensate for such a state of affairs, their graduation could only be granted once all fees had been paid back in settlement but without interest payments required. The Littlejohn family acknowledge that some failed to do so, which added an extra financial burden. It was endured stoically by Littlejohn himself but resented very much by his family.[23] Additionally, the fragile state of the BSO was a major factor in considering its transfer to independent trustees. In 1940, over a celebratory lunch, Littlejohn completed the contracts and by doing so he relinquished not only control but his presence at the school too. Exhortations of support for JML continued right up to the end of his life but the role of Dean had become titular rather than meaningful. However, one further event would bring his influence to bear on who should run the school as de facto head.

By the time a first GCRO directory was published, all opposition led by Hall had dwindled following BSO accreditation. Subsequent register membership within six months had increased the ratio of UK trained full members from parity to 64%:36% in favour of BSO graduates over their BOA counterparts.[24] It fundamentally set the GCRO as a BSO institution for the next four and half decades, to the exclusion of other worthy groups.

Meanwhile Hall's ascendancy as the de facto BSO Dean appeared from the outside as a foregone conclusion. Tommy Hall, a gifted technician, was indebted to his loyal wife Dr Dorothy Wood, who had wholeheartedly involved herself in her husband's professional affairs. She enthusiastically supported the BSO, its students and Littlejohn throughout those tenuous pre-war years. But early in 1940, things began to go wrong.

Hall, venting his feelings with a dramatic gesture, resigned as BSO vice-Dean citing a series of "small incidents over a long period of time".[25] A year beforehand, Littlejohn's frail health had taken a turn for the worse, Shilton Webster-Jones (Webber) and Clem Middleton subsequently had taken on Littlejohn's lecture commitments after his subsequent bouts of ill-health. They were surprised by Hall's refusal to do the same, but it can be surmised that Hall was starting to suffer from hereditary mental problems, especially those of mild paranoia, exacerbated by regular bouts of drinking and his increased dependence on alcohol. At a time when many medical and paramedical people consumed large amounts of alcohol, Hall, like many of us too, succumbed to these traits for the rest of his life. The latter fuelled his paranoia that certain individuals were against him, notably the anti-BSO BOA osteopaths together with Webber and Middleton. His wife Dorothy was to receive alternately his expressions of love when sober but wrath and vitriol when under the influence. She was not helped either by other women attracted to her charismatic, handsome husband.

These episodes were interposed by times of tenderness, conviviality and extreme kindness. Dorothy was no wall-flower accepting these black rages as a dutiful wife. Any woman who had gone through medical school at the time would have had to tolerate a certain level of misogyny and male high jinks. As the marriage went on, Dorothy became less dutiful, while some BSO colleagues such as Webber and Middleton grew more apprehensive about which of Tommy Hall's personalities would appear at any given moment.[26] Others were unaware of his mood swings quite in the same way, beseeching Webber and Middleton to accept his histrionics as Churchillian attributes.[27] The duo had run the BSO diligently throughout the worst period of London bombing and destruction during the Second World War but had decided enough was enough. During 1943, American trained Jocelyn Proby had been contacted by frail Littlejohn to act as his deputy BSO Dean and join its board of governing directors. When Proby found life too onerous in war-torn London, he decided to escape its abrasiveness and strictures to the more gentle Wicklow hills outside Dublin, recommending Hall's appointment as deputy Dean, oblivious of the outcome this decision would cause.

In these circumstances, Webber and Middleton offered their resignations from the BSO faculty, they had had enough of Tommy Hall's black dog outrages. In his letter to the chairman of the BSO board, Webber tries to suggest that this was not a personal criticism of Hall, but indeed for certain it was that, all involved bar Proby knew it too.[28] Furthermore, Webber had been advised by his solicitor not to associate Hall's name with alcohol or schizophrenia.[29] Webber was adamant though, there would be no bargaining or accommodation with Hall's appointment, both he and Middleton would resign their posts instantly. Even Littlejohn pleaded with them both to reconsider their decision and demonstrated proof of improved health by offering to participate more as Dean by supervising Hall's actions. Moreover, he fully expected to visit the school occasionally now that the weather was better.[30] Reading between the lines, Littlejohn does nothing to change Proby's decision reappointing Hall as Vice-Dean. Additionally, Webber knew that JML could no longer cope even as titular, let alone with Hall unleashed as the de facto dean. This drama had a profound consequence on the direction of UK Osteopathy.

A year later, Dorothy Wood would withdraw her commitments and support to the BSO. This was part of her alienation towards osteopathy and eventual divorce from Hall himself. What he could not understand was that his mental instability fuelled by alcohol would devastate any relationship. His second wife and secretary Barbara worked with him from the early 1950s onwards, being very understanding and long-suffering too even until her death in the mid 1980s. Hall finally cut off his association with the BSO in 1964 but was to continue finding expression from teaching and demonstrations as an outstanding technique lecturer and as a well known society osteopath with a practice in the West End. He supported groups outside GCRO influence and laid emphasis on technical wizardry through his friendship with John Wernham and Tom Dummer. To a young graduate, Hall was a decent, supportive, affable and kind elder statesman, but he was a Jekyll and Hyde character in his dealings with the BSO.

In 1947, Littlejohn congratulated Webber on his appointment as BSO vice-Dean and commended him as a wonderful addition to the staff combined with his many years of BSO service. JML's affirmation that Webber was the right person to hand over stewardship to of the BSO should have happened some eight years before.[31] Webber was to take over as BSO Dean, renamed Principal, on Littlejohn's death, a year later. He and Middleton were joined by Audrey Smith (Lady Percival), Margot Gore and Colin Dove, to make up a coherent team to lead the BSO over the next decades. This team worked well, (underpaid and overworked!) so that BSO graduates have played an influential role over UK osteopathy's direction. Colin Dove with other BSO graduates, Stuart Korth and Joyce Vetterlein, ensured that another team headed by Tom Dummer and Margery Bloomfield with Harold Klug, Robert Lever, Jack Taylor, Simon Fielding and Sue Turner of the European School of Osteopathy and its graduates opened the GCRO membership to other alumni, but incisively influenced osteopathy towards a unified profession and statutory regulation.

1. Canning, J. and others to Banbury, H: verification of JML academic awards undated. NOA: scanned Material, J Martin Littlejohn documents. pp.1-2
2. House of Lords Select Committee, *Registration and Regulation of Osteopaths Bill*. London: HMSO, 1935 pp.219-234
3. National Osteopathic Archive: OAGB archive. Incorporated Assocation Osteopaths Volume 2: 1934-36 pp.27-28
4. Hill, C & Clegg, H A, *What is Osteopathy?* London: H Dent & Sons 1937 pp. 128,130, & 182
5. Kennard A & S *Littlejohn family interview* NOA.DVD 2011
6. Littlejohn, J.M., *The Journal of Osteopathy* July-August Volume VII No.4 pp.1-3
7. Hall, T.E., letter *Time &Tide* 25 May 1935 NOA. T E Hall archive. File Box 1
8. Kennard, Anne & Sara, *Littlejohn Family* interview NOA. DVD 2011
9. BOA Council minutes 5 April 1935 pp. 149-150
10. *The Osteopathic Blue Book: Origins and development of Osteopathy in Great Britain* London GCRO pp.24-5
11. ibid pp. 25-7
12. Museum of Osteopathic Medicine, ASO records: Littlejohn school record: J Martin and James Buchan Littlejohn p.314
13. GCRO *The Register of Osteopaths Directory* 1939 p..11
14. Dove, C I, NOA.DVDs. BSO Interview: No.1 2008
15. Museum of Osteopathic Medicine. *2 Littlejohn Brothers*. Correspondence pp.D345.00-345.33
16. Littlejohn J M, travelled prewar to America meeting up with his Uncle James and family NOA. James & Edgar Littlejohn archive. Filebox 1. Trip to USA.
17. NOA. GCRO Council minutes 12 March 1937 pp.77-78. Application came under four headings: BOA- Automatic approval, only group able to sit on council; OAGB; National Society of Osteopaths; and independents, individual associate membership.
18. NOA.GCRO Council minutes pp.78-80
19. NOA.OAGB council minutes 3 October 1936
20. Littlejohn, J. M., Obituary of Ray Harvey Foote, *The Journal of Osteopathy* July- September 1937 Vol. VIII No.3 p.7 & p.10
21. *The Journal of Osteopathy* October- December 1938 Vol. IX No.4 pp.20-21 and April-June 1939 Vol. X No.1 p.11; & pp. 17-20.
22. NOA.GCRO Council minutes p.149
23. Kennard, Anne & Sara, *Littlejohn Family* interview NOA. DVD 2011
24. NOA.GCRO archives: *Analysis of 1939 Register of Members and Associate Members* (1953)
25. Collins, M p.209
26. O'Brien J C, I had many meetings with TEH, he was always a kind, very generous, complimentary person. He encouraged my osteopathic historical interest by donating much of his material in September 1969, which now resides in the NOA archive. He could have made an interesting parent....
27. Canning, J to S J Webster-Jones 11 March 1943 NOA. Quality scanned material. BSO. Disruption 1943. pp.8-10
28. Webster-Jones, S J, to BSO Board 8 March 1943 NOA. Quality scanned material. BSO. Disruption 1943. p.4
29. Blakeney, G, Blakeney & Co., Solicitors to S J Webster- Jones: 26 March 1943: NOA. Quality scanned material. BSO. Disruption 1943. pp.15-16
30. Littlejohn, J. M., personal letters to S J Webster-Jones NOA. Littlejohn Archive. 26 March 1943 pp.1-2
31. Littlejohn, J. M., personal letters to S J Webster-Jones NOA. Littlejohn Archive. 18 April 1947 pp.3-4

Chapter 7

Finale

What do we make of John Martin Littlejohn? A family man whose beloved wife Mabel, and six children (all born in the USA) - Mary, James, Mabel, Edgar, John and Elizabeth (another boy, born on their return to the UK, died prematurely) -seemed close and affectionate towards him and one another too. Yet compare him with his younger brother James. Although they shared many ambitions and goals, other than in their early family life it was James who was more accomplished. The youngest, David, had dabbled with osteopathy but eventually gave it up and went his own way. And a brooding presence over them all was the elder brother, William.

William was at least three years older than J Martin. He seems to have accepted being spectacularly outshone by JML at school. How frustrating for William to find himself enrolled with his brother on the same course at Glasgow University to train for the church. It was JML who became the star academic performer, being offered a living before his brother. Therefore it was William who saw no professional future in Ireland, and was the first member of the family to emigrate to the USA, subsequently followed by his parents and brothers. This powerful vein of ministry within the Littlejohn family was overtaken by a propensity for medicine: William trained as an orthodox MD after a substantial time within the ministry. We know nothing specific of his medical training but we do know that he practised for a considerable time in Michigan.[1] Was it within a reputable establishment or similar to the discredited one attended by David?[2] (Who left the osteopathic profession in 1906 to further a career in public health.) Be that as it may, William veered away from following his brothers into osteopathy.[3]

Returning to J Martin, his early adult career and experience in the Presbyterian Church rendered him legalistic and unswerving, but others might reply that it also made him uncooperative, pedantic and obsessive.[4] His formative years were indeed just that, having a defining lifelong influence on the nature of his character.

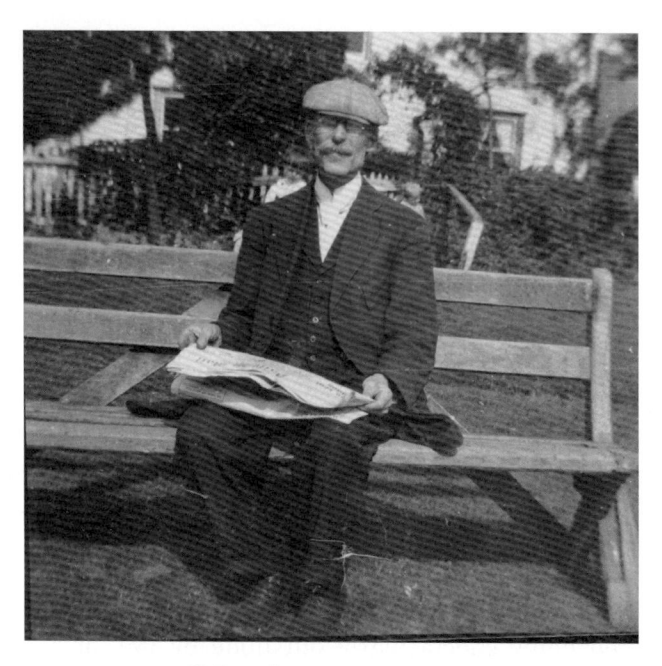

JML in happy retirement

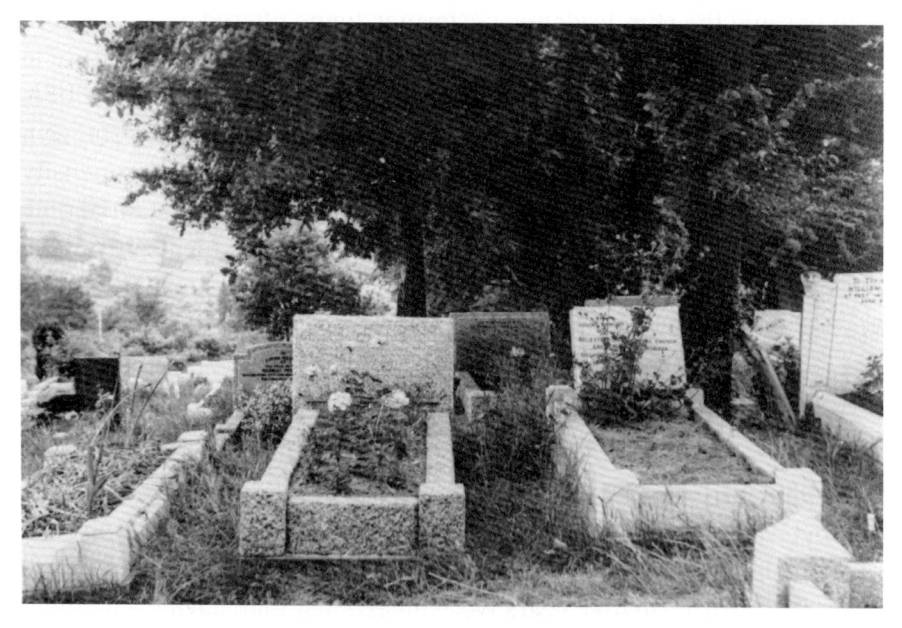

JML's resting place

Philosophical approach

We have steered away from any of J M Littlejohn's writings and books for a number of reasons, but largely due to their impenetrable quality. If anyone needed a copy editor it was JML. Despite his own turgid style, it has to be acknowledged how widely read he was and how his writings appear quite academic but also rather esoteric. His *Principles of Osteopathy* contains 463 pages, being quite unstructured. He continually returns to familiar themes, having strayed to other subjects before resuming to his original text. However, each familiar theme contains a variation of different nuances. His writings describe a universal idea of an individual being integrated within its environment. He differs from A T Still, who expresses a physical element, a 'bone out of place', of structure governing function. Still followed the ideals of the spiritualist Andrew Jackson Davis, the spirit and the physical body as a machine being in harmony, 'created by the free and unobstructed flow of "spirit"'. Any lessening or fluctuations of this force would result in disease.[5] Ultimately, Still's perceptions were interpreted in a narrowly defined osteopathic spinal misplacement, which came under the heading of bodily structure maintaining bodily functions. Littlejohn, on the other hand, endeavours to persuade us that it is function that influences structure, where health is in balance with a number of important factors: structural, obviously, but also environment, mental state, diet and occupation.

Littlejohn's appreciation of health does not emphasise Still's bonesetting principle of malposition causing a lesion either, but he suggests a mal-relationship of the person to structural factors. Ironically, health's opposite is not disease but 'unhealthy'. Littlejohn discusses an interrelationship and interdependence within physiological outcomes as perhaps more pertinent to a person's health rather than pathology or disease. From this standpoint, he intimates that the science of osteopathy is about adjustment to events, one's inability to adjust causes an imbalance to the person's equilibrium and a consequent lowering of the immune system. What osteopathic treatment can do is to eliminate or correct the maladjustment. Here, he perceives the brain and spinal nerves, especially the sympathetic nerves, acting like a vast conduit of pipes or wires which lead to the essential control centres of the body. A very orthodox statement indeed, but Littlejohn's writing style and lack of project planning obscures any true nuggets of information. However, if you are patient enough to continue reading, they are there among the rest.

His language can be flowery when describing physiological or philosophical concepts. Even when he tries to be more specific, its tone becomes increasingly vague and, at times, ends up as waffle. He lacks the clarity and succinctness of his student E S Comstock, or the charisma and oratory of his brother James. However, one cannot ignore homeopathic influences when determining JML's concepts. For five years or so he mixed with some of the best American homeopathic teachers, especially those who adhered to Hahnemann's teachings. It is highly likely that his more multifaceted concept finds resonance in these quarters.

During his time at Kirksville and within osteopathic circles in Chicago, J M Littlejohn's academic abilities overshadowed those of his colleagues. His attempt to found an intellectual journal, *Osteopathic Arena*, failed after its initial run due to a disappointing number of subscribers. Littlejohn's journalism not only suffered from a reputation of dry incomprehensible scholarship, but also his ability to establish a more coherent alternative to A T Still's principle of structure/function and, of course from the unhelpful interfamily litigation which persisted for five years or so.[6]

Aftermath of the BSO

From 1939 onwards Littlejohn no longer taught at the BSO, 16 Buckingham Gate. There were very few students in attendance, but its clinic continued to open. It survived the war years, including the Nazi blitz, but its revenues hardly sustained a fraction of its costs. Consequently the ground floor was rented out to a firm, Bond & Co, and the top floor to Miss Boatman and other rooms as bedsitters too. Meanwhile, the BSO was run by Shilton Webster-Jones (Webber) and Clem Middleton, with the invisible presence of an inquisitive if not inquisitorial T Edward Hall hovering over them from the BSO board. It was inevitable that a major reconstruction of the course and a relaunch of the school were necessary.

In particular, the BSO course was in principle four years long. The first two years were supposed to be attended away from the school building, the assessment rudimentary, variable and, in the main, very basic. The first year contained chemistry, biology and physics up to matriculation level, but many students did not attain this standard. In the second year, anatomy and physiology was taught erratically. Some students were able to go to medical school - Clem Middleton, for example, attended Kings College, which was perfectly adequate. While others made for Chelsea Polytechnic which had a proper anatomy course. But osteopathic students were disadvantaged with no physiology course on offer. Others went to inferior establishments and sat a very substandard BSO exam to gain entry into the third and fourth years. In practical terms, the BSO offered a limited two year course rather than one twice as long. Meanwhile, Middleton and Webber had to plan and effect a curriculum which included a realistic course of a reasonably competent standard to train capable practitioners.

Both realised that the whole course had been dominated by J Martin Littlejohn, and that on reflection his contribution, although influential, was too verbose, with little substance underneath. His lectures were conducted from his reading of his notes or Still's books, a mixture of theology and philosophy. His anatomical mechanics were various diagrams of geometrical lines of forces indicating stresses and strains but never sufficiently practical enough to provide answers. His daily clinical demonstrations on patients were confined to case history taking and a treatment without much of a plan. The case history would involve details of occupation and any trauma suffered, whilst the treatment would combine an appreciation of the state of the superficial body tissues and articulation of specific limb joints leading to the spine. For example, arm pain examination would start at the finger joints and move up the limb inspecting other joints before examining the spine. Littlejohn definitely understood what he was doing but his explanations puzzled many bewildered students. It was hardly a modus operandi that Webber or Middleton could adopt when planning a four year course in the post-war years. Ultimately what did develop (haphazardly) would set UK osteopathy on a path for well over half a century.

In the first three years from 1946 onwards the BSO enrolled a mere 22 students (4, 7 and 11 respectively). Webber based his osteopathic input on the works of Edith Ashmore's *Spinal Mechanics* and Dunning's *Principles of Osteopathy*, two of the most comprehensive osteopathic textbooks of that time. However, clinical hypothesis of specific diagnosis based on the contentious lesion was difficult to define or demonstrate easily. Increasingly alarming was the need to give BSO students, coming from a background perhaps antagonistic to orthodox medicine, a thorough grounding in the basic medical sciences of anatomy, physiology and pathology. Or even expect them to contemplate or understand subjects such as applied anatomy and physiology. To the rescue came someone from a secretarial administrative background, Jessica O'Keefe, who was employed at the BSO as the Principal's secretary.

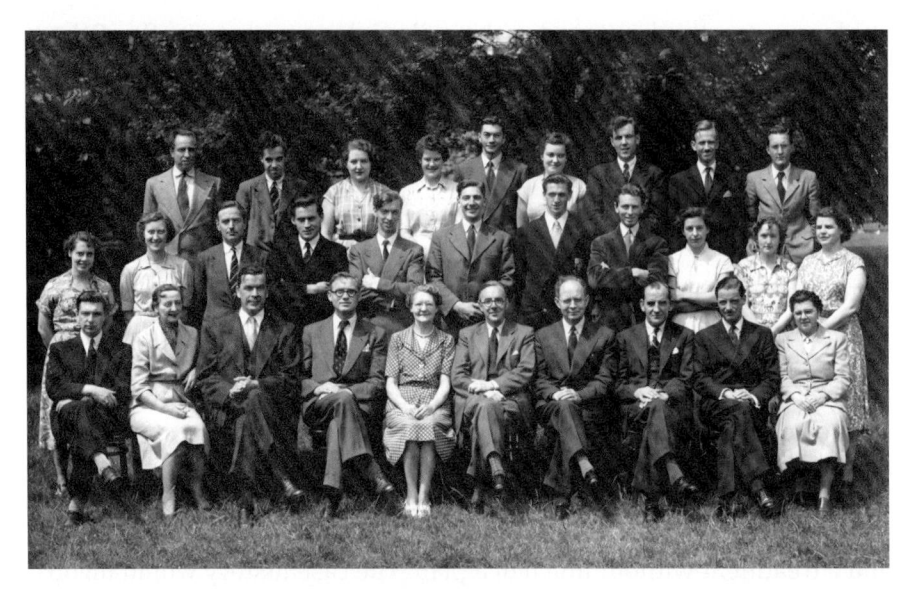

The BSO 1956

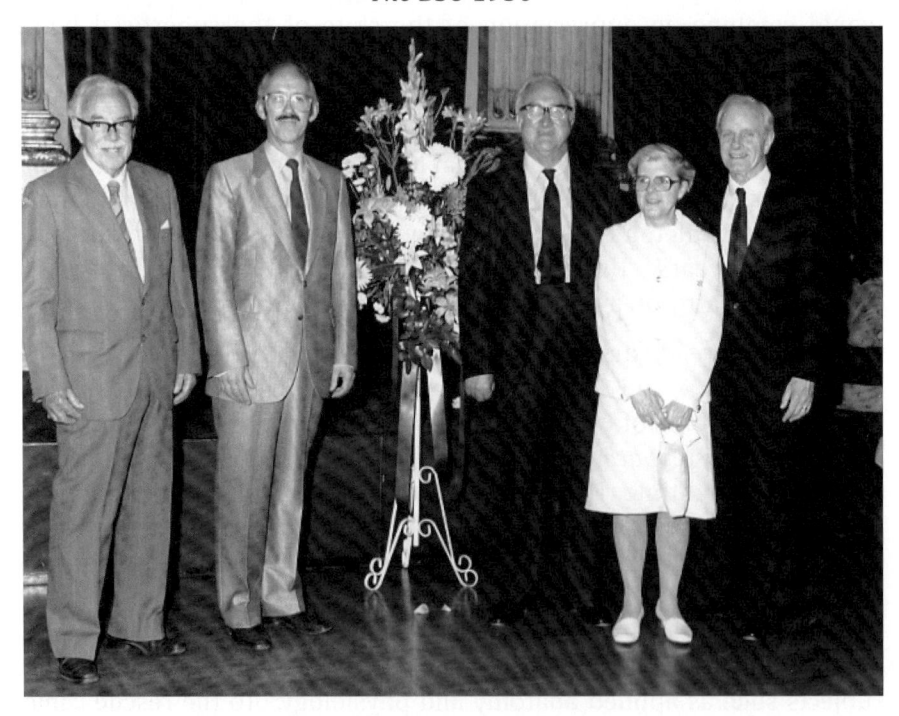

From left to right: Webber, Colin Dove, Stanley Bradford, Audrey, Lady Percival, Sir Norman Lindop

In that position she was well aware of the fragile nature of the BSO finances, its frugal resources and its small student entry. She clearly understood the plight of recruiting suitable staff to teach on an adequate course. She must have had dialogue with Webber and also Middleton, who had struggled together with Muriel Dunning to teach anatomy. Jessica O'Keefe took on an executive role at the BSO, not to the liking of some staff and some governing directors, how dare a non-osteopath and a woman to boot organise our collegiate affairs, was their missive. Jessica O'Keefe rose above these caustic mutterings, she had relayed these conversations to her bright son, Declan, who was studying for his fellowship in Surgery at Guy's Hospital, London. His mother cajoled Declan to volunteer not only to teach anatomy at the BSO but also to extend his contract for three years. A highly strung but temperamental lecturer was Declan O'Keefe. His health was problematical, exacerbated from a persistent peptic ulcer, but he put demobbed servicemen and two female school leavers through an anatomical assault course that would not have been recognised by former BSO alumni or perhaps any other osteopathic teaching institution. He taught it by starting at the back of the chest and going through to the sternum in the front. He would then proceed to do this process from one side to the other. O'Keefe's lectures were three hours long, interspersed by him drinking milk to neutralise his stomach ulcer. Woe betide anyone drifting off, they would feel the lash of his tongue. Students remained conscious of his skills. He turned a motley crew into effective anatomists capable of passing postgraduate medical anatomy exams. His idea of teaching section by section through the body tissues was ideal for osteopathic students as well as aspiring surgical students.

Not finished with his BSO commitment, Declan obtained a friend who was known only by his surname, O'Grady, to teach physiology and another pal, Hugh Pentney, to teach pathology, both from Guy's Hospital. This triumvirate set a standard of teaching of basic medical subjects at the BSO that would lead to improving the teaching of osteopathic subjects as well.[7] However those dissenting BSO directors of Jessica O'Keefe's growing influence were ambivalent about her promotion to a senior management role. They sought to cut her power by initiating a report that criticised her influence and her role.[8] Osteopathy should have congratulated rather than admonish her, for without her contributions the BSO management would have failed dismally.

Meanwhile Webber was a good leader, encouraging others to join the team and being appreciative of their contributions. He was never a great thinker or technician, but his leadership would move the BSO forward through his 21 years as principal. Middleton was always by his side, though without the support from Jessica O'Keefe.

She had left the BSO, not prepared to take such unreasonable criticism, but her involvement had created a tradition whereby anatomy, physiology and pathology were taught to generations of BSO students by medical graduates studying for membership or fellowship exams based at London medical schools. This tradition continued until the school moved from Buckingham Gate to Suffolk Street in the 1980s. Whatever Littlejohn would have made of this we will never know, but Jessica O'Keefe's activity allowed BSO students access to a more balanced training, and the quality of the medical lectures ensured that osteopathic subjects improved too.[9]

After her departure, Webber and Middleton were joined within the inner circle by Audrey Smith (Lady Percival) who had flourished under Declan O'Keefe's tutelage, Margot Gore and Colin Dove. Together they provided a better basis of osteopathic training and were in effect a team of people willing to cooperate in unison for the common good.

Family Life

During the 1930s, the Littlejohn family leased a flat off Baker Street. Weekends were spent out at Badger Hall. From 1939 onwards, J Martin remained most of his time at his country residence. Whether his wife Mabel used the London flat at all is not known, but at Badger Hall she not only held the household together but was rumoured to have run a small school in the grounds. John Wernham, whose parents also lived in the village of Thundersley, may have been one of those attending. In any case, he thought of himself as part of the Littlejohn family with a strong affection for both Mabels, mother and daughter, together with awe for JML. Although J Martin's presence was felt within the house, he would settle in his study as a place of refuge, only appearing at meal times. The dining room was in full view of the driveway, so any person venturing up might have spied the slight figure of J Martin through the French windows hurriedly returning back to the comfortable solitude of his study nearby.[10]

It is suggested by the family that in true Scottish nonconformist tradition the children were influenced by their father's directive concerning specific career moves. Mary and James would go to medical school, Edgar and John to the BSO to train as osteopaths. Mary and Mabel are registered as having attended the BSO together but whether they finished the course has never been established. Little is known of Elizabeth's training, but Mary appears to have dropped out of medical school after two years for some reason. James seems to have done well at St. George's medical school in Knightsbridge, making further advances as an ear, nose and throat surgeon. Edgar, who was his father's favourite, and John were very much reluctant BSO graduates, but both assisted their father at his Dover Street practice. Additionally, Edgar was made BSO vice-Dean for a while until he decided to terminate his osteopathic career in order to run a cycle shop in neighbouring Benfleet. In 1943 Edgar joined the Royal Corps of Signals, and died in India. It is said that J Martin never got over Edgar's death and rather lost the will to continue himself. Son John, a shy diffident individual, on the other hand carried on practising osteopathy in Great Cumberland Place until his retirement in the early 1960s. His family suggest that he never wanted to participate or take a leadership role in the profession. Osteopathy and the BSO did arise from time to time during Littlejohn family conversation during meals, of course, and so his family are of the opinion that he would have been much happier going into business instead.[11]

Some of JML's children rather resented their father's charity towards BSO students delaying or never repaying their BSO fees at the expense of financial sacrifices made by the family. But without his financial assistance to individual students and paying regular administrative costs, the BSO enrolment would probably have been reduced to 3 or 4 students per year and its very existence in severe jeopardy. Also, randomly speculated by the family was the perplexing question as to who would take over as BSO dean after dad? The family felt that the flamboyant T E Hall was a bit of a rake and Webber disappointingly was not popular enough to fulfil such a role. Their father had proposed Jocelyn Proby, (from a well-to-do Northamptonshire family, had all the correct credentials) in 1943 to take over as acting dean. However Proby did not relish wartime curbs of rationing and he decided to escape the deprivations of war-torn London for the relative safety and abundance of Southern Ireland. Surely too, Edgar's and John's lack of interest in the

BSO plus the premature death of Ray Harvey Foote made the decision even harder for Littlejohn to make.

Another awkward subject that was discussed by his children and their descendants was churchgoing family attendance. During their time at Badger Hall, Littlejohn would preach occasionally at the local Congregational chapel and the neighbouring parish church. The whole family were made to attend under sufferance. In his latter years, even though JML stopped attending church, his Christian message in limited osteopathic articles and letters was as strong as ever.[12]

His final years were filled with the sound of grandchildren. They remember a little frail man in a dishevelled suit and a flat cap appearing occasionally for meals. He was amused by and patient with them, but too much noise and frenetic display would be cautioned with the phrase, "all this monkey business about!!"[13]

What of his family in America? His son James made a trip to the USA in 1938 with his father's blessing and met up with uncles William and David together with their respective families. However, his uncle James's family was for some reason excluded, the rupture between J Martin and James still too raw even after three decades. It is good to know that there was a family reunion in the 1990s in Chicago which included James's grandchildren and those of JML which appeared to lay to rest the unpleasant episode between the two grandfathers some eighty years earlier.

JML seemed to harbour a stoical attitude to events in his life, from his problems as a young minister in Northern Ireland to his misadventure in the House of Lords select committee sessions. Outwardly he shrugged off his setbacks.[14]

What can we make of his life and times? He emigrated to the USA for a better life, as so many from Europe were doing at the time, during an exciting period in its history, characterised by the dominance of the northern and north-eastern industrial States and a purposeful national drive to evangelise all things American. Osteopathy had its birth in the backdrop of an attritional Civil War three decades before, its influence spreading to new cities located in the Midwestern States founded by the wholesale misappropriation of native lands and destruction of the indigenous peoples. From this beginning, J Martin Littlejohn spent most of his time in the great cities of New York and Chicago, his vision of osteopathy being inevitably more expansive than A T Still due to his theological and homeopathic background. On returning to Britain his contribution to European osteopathy has been magnificent if rather less coherent than some of us would have wished. Lack of clarity in his writings have allowed others to advance their own interpretations of Littlejohn, but as Professor Stephen Tyreman notes, the gold nuggets are there among the residue. In the end, using a slight ecclesiastical notion, his life, like the curate's egg, was good in parts.

---

1   Kennard, Anne & Sara *Littlejohn family interview* NOA. DVD 2011;
2   Grigg, E R N, *Peripatetic Pioneer: William Smith MD DO (1862-1912)* Journal of the History of Medicine April 1967 p.173
    "David Littlejohn graduated from the Central Medical College in St Joseph's, Missouri, November 1898- a diploma mill."
3   The Chicago College of Osteopathic Medicine (CCOM) inadvertently has placed on their walls a large picture of William and his two children with staff outside his surgery. NOA /quality scanned/American schools/CCOM/Littlejohn/William: *William and his two children plus staff, outside his clinic.*
4   Campbell, C. J M Littlejohn, Early years 4th NOA History Society Symposium: *J Martin Littlejohn* DVD 19th June 2011
5   Gevitz N. *The DO's: Osteopathic Medicine in America* The John Hopkins University Press 1982 p.13
6   Tyreman, S. J M Littlejohn, Philosophical concepts. 4th NOA History Society Symposium: *J Martin Littlejohn* DVD 19th June 2011
7   Audrey Lady Percival, BSO: The post war years 6th NOA History Society Symposium: *History of the BSO* DVD 3 December 2011
8   Report of subcommittee to consider and define the office of principal and duties attaching to that office: part of which was to curb the power held by Mrs O'Keefe, principal's secretary 1954 NOA/BSO/board meetings/filebox9/0704
9   Percival, Lady Audrey *Conversations* March-June 2014
10 Kennard, Anne & Sara *Littlejohn family interview* NOA. DVD 2011
11 Ibid.
12 Ibid.
13 Ibid.
14 Ibid.

Addendum

Before we conclude this study of J Martin Littlejohn, special mention should be made of his writings. There will be others who will concentrate on and interpret them in careful detail, but my task is to prioritise his books and lecture notes rather than his many articles.

We know that he had written a dissertation *The Sabbatism of Hebrews IV: 9* in 1891 that rewarded him with the Henderson Fellowship Theology prize in Glasgow as part of his Bachelor of Divinity degree. This thesis was probably recycled for his Doctor of Divinity from the Night University, Chicago as *"The Christian Sabbatism"*(1894).[1] We have no evidence that this document still exists. However there are a number of copies of his next dissertation, *The Political Theory of Schoolmen,* in existence. What was the point of his printing this incomplete thesis?

Following a successful year as principal of Amity College and his Doctor of Divinity award, JML's next mission was to prepare his unfinished dissertation for submission for a dubious Doctorate of Philosophy from the Night University, Chicago rather than from Columbia College.[2] Indeed, he acknowledges his Colombian College supervisor for his valuable assistance:

"Dr. W. A. Dunning, of Columbia College, to whom I owe grateful thanks for his constant suggestions in the course of the preparation of the Thesis, has carefully gone over all the materials, and on behalf of the Faculty of Political Science has accorded the work his approval as my Doctoral Thesis. To him and the other Members of the Faculty of Political Science in conjunction with my Alma Mater I dedicate this contribution."[3]

JML is endeavouring to portray ambiguously that he successfully completed his PhD under the auspices of Columbia without qualifying whether the Faculty of Political Science and his *Alma Mater* specified is Columbia College or the Night University, Chicago, the difference between the academic standard of each establishment being vast beyond comparison. It's hardly feasible that Dunning ever set eyes on the printed version either, but it did have a restorative role in providing seemingly undisturbed academic progress on JML's curriculum vitae.

This metaphorical lifeboat of the Night University not only provided succour, but also two years later and subsequently, it provided the foundations of his medical training.

Meanwhile, the American School of Osteopathy (ASO) faculty members were encouraged to write books covering their lectures on their specific subjects. Accreditation as a medical school exponentially increased student recruitment to an extent that cohorts of students studied in batches rather than as a whole, due to lack of room to physically accommodate such numbers. Publishing the content of their lectures allowed lecturers to place an osteopathic spin on each subject, it provided a focus for the students inconvenienced by the logistical overcrowding, and it contributed further income for the Still family. Plagiarism was a familiar word in common parlance within academia in the mid-20th century onwards but not in the late 19th century. Particularly in the American Midwest, copying someone else's work would not have been considered untoward. JML's first book was *Physiology: Exhaustive and Practical- A Series of Practical Lectures delivered from Day to Day* (1898).[4]

Much was made of JML's title of "Professor of Physiology" by Sir William Jowitt, BMA Counsel, in the House of Lords select committee hearing.. Jowitt remonstrated with JML for utilising such a title and teaching physiology without having any qualifications in the subject.[5] (Jowitt, educated at Oxford, would have been familiar with the title "professor" related to esteemed Chairs, but in other countries such as the USA, the term can denote merely a lecturer). JML protested that he had studied science, including the subjects of chemistry and elementary physiology under Professor McKendrick at Glasgow University, plus further study in anatomy and physiology at Anderson's Medical School too, although this cannot be substantiated.[6] Elementary physiology was explained lucidly by Thomas Huxley in his popular book, *Lessons in Elementary Physiology*, and it is fitting that this essential material covered what was taught by JML at Kirksville.[7]

JML's second book, *PsychoPhysiology* (1899), was completed at a time of deteriorating relations between the Still Family and the remaining ASO faculty who opposed Bill Smith and the Littlejohn brothers. It is intriguing that JML made some precise connection between psychology and physiology, indeed, he is proud to verify his ASO professorial title of Physiology and Psychology.[8] This was followed by a thirty page booklet, *Osteopathy Explained: The Science of Osteopathy* (1900).

JML had written for *The Journal of the Science of Osteopathy* (February 1900), this unabridged version, *The Science of Osteopathy: Its Value in Preventing and in Curing Disease*. It was delivered in a lecture on the 19th July 1899 to the Society of Science, Letters and Arts at Crystal Palace library, South London. But not at the distinguished Royal Society nor delivered at the Crystal Palace itself (see Chapter 3).[9] This incident was mentioned in a letter by Charlie Still to a Dr. Ernest Roberts, complaining of JML's behaviour in lauding his own lecture and gaining so much free publicity. All this was part of the animosity engendered between the Still and Littlejohn families following the latter's departure from Kirksville and their setting up a rival school in Chicago.[10] Once JML moved to the Illinois city, he continued to lecture and write on other osteopathic subjects.

His lectures on *Practice of Osteopathy* (1901) were typewritten and compiled into a folder to be handed out to students. His notes on *Osteopathic Obstetric Mechanics* (15 February 1902) were published in *The Journal of the Science of Osteopathy*. His *Principles of Osteopathy* were compiled over a number of years and co-authored with Laurence S. Meyran at some stage, comprising of 432 closely typed pages. Similarly, *Osteopathic Therapeutic Diagnosis* consists of the same format of 440 typewritten pages. and acts as a compendium of various osteopathic manipulative procedures for specific diseases and syndromes.

Apart from single-handedly teaching osteopathic related subjects at the British School of Osteopathy for almost two decades, his lecture notes are held in the National Osteopathic Archive. For almost a decade he edited and wrote continuously in *the Journal of Osteopathy* up to the outbreak of the Second World War.

1   Littlejohn J M, JM Littlejohn archive NOA scanned material. *The Political Theory of Schoolmen.* May 1895 pp.2-3.
2   Grant E J , Registrar, Columbia University Letter to Professor F J Fordyce, Glasgow University. 29 July 1942:outlining JML's major subject of study, political philosophy , for his PhD but the absence of "his name from the listings of recipients of that degree".
3   Littlejohn J M, *The Political Theory of Schoolmen* Preface. May 1895.
4   Littlejohn J M *Physiology: Exhaustive and Practical- A Series of Practical Lectures delivered from Day to Day* Journal Printing Company. 1898. Title page.
5   House of Lords Select Committee, *Registration and Regulation of Osteopaths Bill.* London: HMSO, 1935 p.229:3472-3488.
6   bid p.230: 3497.
7   Huxley, Thomas H. *Lessons in Elementary Physiology* MacMillan, London 1870 fourth edition
8   Littlejohn J M, *PsychoPhysiology* E G Kinney, Kirksville, Mo., 1899 title page.
9   Littlejohn J M, *The Science of Osteopathy: Its Value in Preventing and in Curing Disease* (1900)
10 Still, CE to E Roberts, a copy of letter: complaining of JML's behaviour 23 March 1900

Index

Adamson MP, W M: 74
Addran (Adranx) Christian University, Waco, Texas: 17, 20
American College of Osteopathic Medicine & Surgery: 42
American Medical Association: 69, 77
American Osteopathic Association: 60, 63, 68, 92
American School of Osteopathy, Kirksville : 23-4, 26, 30, 32, 34-5, 42, 48, 53, 61
Amity College, Iowa: 16, 18-9, 29, 34, 40
Anderson, George: 77, 80-1
Ashmore, Edith: 105
A T Still Research Institute: 55
Axham, W F: 59

Badger Hall, Benfleet, Essex: 57-8, 73, 89, 92, 95-6, 109
Barker, Sir Herbert: 58-61, 67, 75-6, 88
Bishoff, Fred: 48
Boatman, Miss: 104
Bonesetters: 58-60
Boothby MP, Robert: 74, 76
Bradford, Stanley: 106
British College of Chiropractic: 64
British Medical Association: 64, 76-8, 80-1
British Osteopathic Association: 61-3, 65, 67-9, 73-5, 78, 87, 91, 93-6
British Osteopathic Society (precursor of British Osteopathic Association): 59-60
British School of Osteopathy: 50, 55, 58, 61-9, 73, 75, 78, 84, 87-98, 104-109
Buxton MP, Noel: 60

Calvinism: 15
Cathcart, Thomas: 9
Central Michigan Medical School: 30
Charteris, Matthew: 13
Chesterton, Mrs: 80, 82-3, 91
Chicago College of Osteopathy: 62
Chiropractic (US): 68, 77
Coleraine Academical Institute: 6
Collins, Martin: 16
Columbia College, New York: 15-6, 18, 53
Comstock, Ernest S: 45, 48
Cook County Hospital, Chicago: 47
Cooper, William: 61
Creevagh, Ireland: 8-12, 17

Dawson, Lord: 80, 83-4
Denslow, Steadman: 44
Dickens, Hal: 80
Dove, Colin: 93, 99, 106, 108
Dummer, Thomas: 99
Dunham Homeopathic Medical School: 19-20, 33, 41-3, 45, 55
Dunham, Jay: 55
Dunning, Muriel: 65
Dunning, William R: 15, 18

Elibank, Viscount: 78, 84, 92

European School of Osteopathy, Maidstone: 99
Fielding, Simon: 99
Fink, Charles: 48
Flexner, Abraham: 27, 43, 46-8, 69, 94
Foote, Ray Harvey: 55, 63, 78, 80, 87-88, 92, 95-6, 109
Forbes, Mary (Bill Smith's sister in law): 34

Garvagh, Northern Ireland: 4, 5, 13
Garvagh Academy: 5-7
General Council and Register of Osteopaths:91-2, 94-7, 99
General Medical Council: 58-60, 76
Glasgow University: 6-7, 14, 29, 53-4, 101
Gore, Margot: 99
Green, Wilfred: 78
Greenwood MP, Arthur: 75
Grotius, Hugo: 15-17

Hahnemann Homeopathic Medical College, Chicago: 42
Hall, Thomas Edward: 53, 66, 91, 94, 96-9, 104
Hamilton, Warren: 39
Hawthorn, C O: 77
Hazzard, Charles: 29, 32, 37
Hempson, Oswald A: 77-78, 80-1
Hering Homeopathic Medical School, Chicago: 19, 33, 42-3, 45, 55
Hill, Charles: 77, 81
Horn, Franz: 55, 61
Hough, Clara: 58
Hough Collins, Mrs J E: 58
Houston T G: 6
Hudson Dr: 60
Hulett C M T: 27, 33

Huxley, Thomas: 29-30
Illinois State Board of Health: 19, 46-7, 49, 94
Incorporated Association of Osteopaths (*precursor of Osteopathic Association of Great Britain*): 63-4, 67-9, 73-5, 87-8
Irish Nationalism: 8-9
Jowitt, Sir William: 16, 29, 53, 78-83, 87-8

Kaiser Frederick III: 13
Kent, James Tyler: 41
Kirksville College of Osteopathic Medicine: 67
Klug, Harold: 99
Korr, Irwin: 44
Korth, Stewart: 99

Laughlin, George M (*Blanche Still's husband*): 40-1
Lever, Robert: 99
Lindop, Sir Norman: 106
Ling, Per: 32, 37
Littlejohn, Buchan (brother-deceased in childhood): 1
Littlejohn College of Osteopathy, Chicago: 45-9, 55, 93
Littlejohn, David (*brother*): 2, 19-20, 26, 29-41, 43, 45, 53, 101
Littlejohn, Edgar (*JML's son*):73, 89-90, 101, 109
Littlejohn, Edith Mary (*James Buchan's wife*): 45, 49, 56-7, 94
Littlejohn, Elizabeth (JML's *mother*): 1, 3, 46, 54-5, 57
Littlejohn, Elizabeth (*JML's daughter*): 101, 109
Littlejohn, Elizabeth Alexander (*sister*): 2, 41

Index

Littlejohn, James (JML's *father*): 1-5, 8, 11-3, 34, 55
Littlejohn, James (*JML's son*): 89-90, 93-4, 101, 109
Littlejohn, James Buchan (*brother*): 2, 12, 14, 18, 20, 26, 29-30, 32-9, 41, 43, 45, 49, 53, 55-7, 93-4, 101, 104, 109
Littlejohn, Janet Elizabeth (*sister-deceased in childhood*): 2
Littlejohn, John Martin: Schools and Glasgow University 1, 4-8; Ministry at Garvagh, Northern Ireland 8-13; Further Glasgow University 14, Columbia College, New York 15-6; Night National University (National Medical College) Chicago 16-20, 23, 29, 40-1, 53; Amity College, Iowa 18; Kirksville, Missouri 23, 26, 29-37; Chicago 39-50, 55-7, 62; degrees and doctorates: 53-54; Return to UK 58; British School of Osteopathy 61-8, 87-97; House of Lords Select Committee 73-5,78-84; Finale 101-5,109-110.
Littlejohn, John Martin Junior (*JML's son*): 89-90, 93, 101, 109
Littlejohn, Mabel (*JML's wife*): 41, 45, 54, 56-7, 101, 108
Littlejohn, Mabel (*JML's daughter*): 101, 109
Littlejohn, Margaret (sister-deceased in childhood): 2
Littlejohn, Mary (*JML's daughter*): 101, 108-109
Littlejohn, William (*brother*): 2, 4, 6, 12-3, 40, 46, 56-7, 101

Looker, William (Looker School of Osteopathy & Chiropractic, Manchester): 63-4, 81
Lorimer, Sir James: 15
Lowber Dr: 17
Lowry, Gerald: 62

MacDonald, Kelman: 61-2, 76-8, 80-1, 83, 87-8, 91-2, 95-6
MacKenzie, Sir Morrell: 13
Maxwell, Mary: 81
McConnell, Carl: 29, 32, 37, 40, 48
McKendrick, J G: 14
Mennell, James: 75
Middleton, Clem: 65, 97-8, 104-5, 107-8
Miller, W G: 15
Milne, Herbert: 95
Ministry of Health: 67
Moore, Henry: 90
Moore, J Stewart: 58, 61
Murphy, Harold: 81

Night National University (National Medical College) Chicago 16-20, 23, 29, 40-1, 53

O'Keefe, Declan: 107
O'Keefe, Jessica (*mother*): 105, 107-8
O'Grady, Dr: 107
Osteopaths Bill (1935) House of Lords Select committee: 1, 16,19, 29, 53, 64, 69, 76-9, 81-4, 87, 93, 109
Osteopathic Association of Great Britain: 88, 92, 94-5
Osteopathic Defence League: 60, 67, 69, 74-6, 79-80, 88

Palmer B J (*son*): 27
Palmer D D (*Father*): 27

119

Percival, Audrey, Lady (*nee Smith*): 99, 106, 108
Pheils, Elmer: 63
Poole, Reginald G: 15-16
Proby, Jocelyn: 98, 109
Proctor, C W: 29, 32, 37
Proctor, Ernest: 48

Quimby, Phineas Parkhurst: 36

Reformed Presbyterian Church: 2-6, 8, 20, 101.
Reformed Presbyterian Church, Southern Presbytery & Moderator: 10-12
Roman Catholic Church: 12
Royal Society: 42. 54
Royal Society of Literature: 41-2, 54

St. Joseph's, Central Michigan College: 40
Saul, Pat: 95
St. Joseph's Missouri: 40
Seaton, Elwyn D: 19
Shaw, George Bernard: 63
Smith, William (Bill): 23-7, 32-7
Society of Science, Letters & Arts: 32, 42, 53-5
Stephens, Lou: 26
Still, Andrew Taylor: 23-7, 30-4, 36-8, 40, 44-5, 47, 68, 77, 93, 103, 105-6, 110
Still, Blanche (*daughter*): 28, 40

Still, Charlie (*son*): 28, 33-5, 38, 42, 54
Still, Fred (*son*): 28
Still, Harry (*son*): 28-9, 3-34, 38-40
Still, Hermon (*son*): 28
Stoddard, Alan: 65
Streeter, Wilfrid: 60-1, 74-6, 78-80, 83, 88, 92
Swengel, Flora: 45

Taylor, Jack: 99
Thomson, Sir William (Lord Kelvin): 13
Thorpe, J H: 79, 84
Turner, Sue: 99
Tyreman, Stephen: 110

University of Chicago: 16

Van Straten: 95

Vetterlein, Joyce: 99

Walker, Willard: 55
Wareing, Elsie: 62
Waukesha Sanatorium: 16-17
Webster-Jones, Shilton (*Webber*): 63, 65, 97-9, 104-8
Wernham, J: 99, 108
Western School of Osteopathy, Plymouth: 64
Whiting, C A: 55
Wood, Dorothy (*T E Hall's wife*): 95-9